SKIN DEEP

*The Real Truth About Beauty,
Aging, and Skincare That Works*

GIN AMBER

Skin Deep
The Real Truth About Beauty, Aging, and Skincare That Works

ginamber.com

Copyright © 2026 Gin Amber

All rights reserved
No portion of this book may be reproduced mechanically, electronically, or by any other means, including photocopying, without securing the advanced written permission of the author. Likewise, no portion of this book may be posted to a website or distributed by any other means without securing the advanced written permission of the author.

Limits of liability and disclaimer of warranty
This book is strictly for informational and educational purposes only. Neither the author nor the publisher shall be liable for any misuse of the enclosed material. The author and the publisher do not guarantee that anyone following these techniques, suggestions, tips, ideas, or strategies will be successful or healed. The author and the publisher shall have neither liability nor responsibility to anyone with respect to any loss or damage caused, or alleged to be caused, directly or indirectly, by the information or suggestions contained in this book.

Medical disclaimer
To the extent that any medical or health information is shared in this book, it is provided as an information resource only and is not to be used or relied on for any diagnostic or treatment purposes. Any such information does not constitute patient information, does not create any patient-physician relationship, and should not be used as a substitute for professional diagnosis and treatment.

Published by Made to Change the World™ Publishing
Nashville, Tennessee

ISBN: 978-1-956837-71-1 (print)
ISBN: 978-1-956837-72-8 (ebook)

Printed globally.

To you—

The woman standing in front of the mirror wondering
when her skin stopped feeling like her own.

The one who's fought silent battles—
with aging, with acne, with shame, with doubt.

The one who's tried every cream, every trick,
every promise, and still feels unseen.

The one suffering from the sting of insecurity,
the confusion of misinformation,
and the desperate search for something real.

This book is for you.

I see you.
I feel you.
I was you.

You are not alone in this.

Let this be the moment you stop chasing perfection
and start reclaiming your power—skin, soul, and self.

CONTENTS

Foreword 1

Acknowledgments 3

Introduction 5

Chapter 1: Beauty & Self-Love 11

Chapter 2: Understanding Skincare Basics 25

Chapter 3: The Psychology of Beauty 35

Chapter 4: Building a Skincare Routine 45

Chapter 5: Chronic Skin Issues 57

Chapter 6: Promoting Healthy Skin from the Inside . . . 65

Chapter 7: Skincare through the Ages 75

Chapter 8: Microneedling and Dermarolling 83

Chapter 9: Additional Skincare Tools 99

A Note from Me to You 107

About the Author 109

Frequently Asked Questions 111

FOREWORD

For more than two decades, I've dedicated my scientific career to unlocking the power of nitric oxide, one of the most important molecules produced in the human body, which controls the regulation of blood flow and oxygen to every organ, tissue, and cell. My research, the scientific questions I address, and the discoveries I have made have always been with a solution in mind. One of my most innovative scientific breakthroughs is the topical nitric oxide technology. It not only compensates for the body's declining ability to produce nitric oxide, but it helps restore the body's ability to naturally produce it again, delivering it directly where it matters most.

But beyond the science, I bring a deeply human perspective to skincare. I've seen how aging isn't just about numbers or surface wrinkles—it's about vitality, resilience, and connection. That's why skincare has always been more than a cosmetic endeavor to me. It's a bridge between inner health and outer well-being. Our skin reflects our systemic health.

So when I first met Gin Amber and experienced her approach, I was struck by how genuinely aligned she is with this vision. She doesn't chase trends. She educates. She simplifies complex biology into actionable insight. Her philosophy—that nitric oxide isn't magic, but rather the body's language for healing and renewal—is the same I have held. We both firmly believe that optimal skincare is about providing the body with the tools it's already wired to use.

That's what makes *Skin Deep* so rare and necessary. It doesn't just rehash the same skincare cliches. Gin speaks to topics that matter—microneedling, the biological underpinnings of aging, nutrition's role in skin repair, and holistic healing rooted in evidence. She takes you beyond quick fixes. She helps you rebuild your skincare philosophy from the inside out.

What you will gain from this book goes far beyond topical skincare routines. You'll gain perspective. A shift in how you view self-care—not as a surface act, but as a deliberate practice in honoring your body's innate intelligence. You'll learn to trust science that's been tested and peer-reviewed, not unchecked hype or exaggerated marketing claims.

In a world where beauty is often packaged with profit-first agendas and superficial promises, Gin's work shines through with clarity and integrity. I'm proud to endorse this book and her brand because it represents a different path—one where science, healing, and authenticity guide the conversation.

If you're ready to embrace a skincare journey anchored in biology, respect, and real results, this is the book for you. It's not just about looking younger— it's about helping your body do what it already knows how to do: heal, rejuvenate, and flourish. And I'm confident this will transform not just your skin, but the way you care for yourself.

Nathan S. Bryan, Ph.D.
Inventor, Author, Scientist, Entrepreneur

ACKNOWLEDGMENTS

To my incredible community—thank you. This book, and everything it stands for, wouldn't exist without you. To every follower who liked a video, left a comment, sent a message, or shared their story—you gave me the courage to keep going. Your trust, your questions, and your transformations have been my greatest inspiration.

To all the people who felt lost in the sea of skincare advice, overwhelmed by contradicting voices, and discouraged by products that overpromised and underdelivered—this book is for you.

Thank you to the holistic health professionals, dermatologists, plastic surgeons, estheticians, and researchers who shared your time, knowledge, and insights over the years. You helped deepen my understanding of the body-skin connection and inspired me to ask better questions. Special thanks to the books, studies, and thought leaders that helped me uncover the truth and protect others from harm.

To my team at Gin Amber Beauty—I'm so grateful for your passion, dedication, and shared belief that beauty should never come at the cost of health. Thank you for standing behind my vision and helping me deliver toxic-free, education-driven skincare to people around the world.

To the pioneers of clean beauty, to the skeptics who made me research harder, and to every soul searching for answers beyond the surface—I honor you.

And finally, to anyone who has ever stared into the mirror and wondered why nothing seems to work, who's tired of guessing what's right or safe for their skin—you're not alone. You deserve answers rooted in truth, not trends. You deserve skincare that heals, not hides. You deserve to feel safe, confident, and radiant in your own skin.

Thank you for trusting me to guide you there.

INTRODUCTION

I've always been fascinated by skin. What serves as the barrier between the most intimate and vulnerable parts of yourself and the world around you is a matter of millimeters—the power of life at the mercy of this incredible design. Skin is an artform, a medium that tells your stories in the most private way: a smile line here, a scar there, a reminder of the place where your children entered the world... Your skin is the story of you.

For centuries, even millennia, people have been defined according to their skin. The color of skin has launched wars and brought entire kingdoms to their knees. Who you were, what you were allowed to do with your life, who you loved, and what you had access to often was determined by your skin. This skin that humanizes you, that holds you together, that shares details of your story with everyone you meet without uttering a word. *This is who I am; this is what I have endured; this is my history, my culture, my pain, my joy.* This skin is my declaration: *I am here; I am allowed to take up space in this world. See me.*

And yet this organ that protects everything you are is so misunderstood. Your skin acts like a messenger, sending signals about what's going on inside your body. When you're not balanced, your skin will show you signs. Yet, rather than listen, nurture, and provide for its needs, perhaps you try to punish your skin into healing. Hasn't this become the message of the modern world? Do more, be more, buy more, fix more. Beauty products overpromise and underdeliver, and your skin absorbs the impact. Can you hear what your skin is trying to tell you? Or are you both starved and overwhelmed with excess at the same time—flooded with skincare trends and short-term advice when all you're truly looking for is honesty and uncomplicated beauty. While you want to embody your instinctive power to care for your own skin sustainably and authentically, you instead get noise and mixed messages. The result is a cluttered beauty industry that does little for the average woman's skin.

Now, there is nothing wrong with beauty trends or cosmetics (and I'm a firm believer in balance and doing what feels right for your unique skincare needs), so I'm not advocating for boycotting the beauty trends or products you love. I'm not advocating for radical change or complex routines. What I'm offering is the opposite: a simplification, a refining of all that you know and all that you do down to the most essential advice about how to give yourself the skin you deserve.

Growing up in a small Lithuanian village of just five thousand people, my childhood was simple and community-focused. But as peaceful as this was, I wasn't free from the insecurities that most girls face in childhood. Like so many girls, my self-worth was fragile, and I constantly compared myself to others. I lacked confidence, particularly about my appearance, and felt that my acne and rosacea meant that I was ugly and unlovable. Over the next two decades, my skin would become an all-consuming issue that eventually led me to a place of destruction and rebirth—the desperation that became the foundation for Gin Amber Beauty.

In my twenties, I moved to Miami in search of *more*. I wanted more growth, more freedom, more opportunities. But I brought my insecurities with me. Even at my tender age, I was already experiencing premature aging

INTRODUCTION

lines, dark circles under my eyes, and dilated blood vessels. Miami was a foreign world compared to my small village; a vibrant and diverse city with impossibly high beauty standards that I felt intense pressure to meet. I used alcohol to try to numb my increasing anxiety about the way I looked, which, of course, only fed a vicious cycle. The more I drank to escape my negative feelings about myself, the worse my overall health—including my skin health—became. Eventually, I was battling many skin and health issues while living in a city that seemed to prioritize perfection, which only made my struggles worse.

I don't think I'm alone in my experience of the struggles and insecurities I've had with my skin or my obsession with perfection. This is the modern dilemma, the highest form of self-abuse: procuring perfection—no matter the cost. The insecurities come in many forms: wrinkles, stretch marks, hyperpigmentation, scars, or acne. Whatever issue you're facing, this truth is universal: Your skin is what the world sees first. And while I don't believe that it should be this way, the reality is that first impressions are made based on the way that you look.

So I spent decades pursuing this shallow, externally-derived sort of satisfaction—with myself, my appearance, my place in the world. And in the end, it cost me all of those things.

My journey of transformation began when I started seeking something deeper. I knew that what I was chasing would never be satisfied with shallow pursuits. I knew that the way I felt about myself—the lack of self-love and compassion for my own suffering—was being reflected back at me through my skin.

My struggles took me to an emotional space that allowed me to start seeing my life through the lens of authenticity and self-love. Books like *The Gifts of Desperation* helped me understand that living a life rooted in love and service—not external validation—was the key to true peace and fulfillment.

One particular quote from *The Gifts of Desperation* has always stayed with me:

> *I am always happy inside, no matter what life throws at me. Serving the Creator's desire for me fills my heart with pure joy. Watching others gain hope and inspiration excites my soul and motivates me to keep going.*

This wisdom resonated deeply with me at a time in my life when I was craving purpose and belonging. It helped give me the clarity I needed to let go of my pursuit for perfection and find approval within myself. As I healed the wounds within that others couldn't see, slowly my skin began to heal too. I realized the connection between emotional and mental health and skin health, and this became a source of strength for me. I embraced the lessons life was teaching me through my pain and experienced an awakening. I stopped drinking alcohol and began questioning everything, from the societal norms and beauty standards I had internalized to the ingredients in my skincare products.

This journey has given me the power to empathize with other women who are facing the heartbreak and isolation that skin conditions can cause and has inspired me to guide and equip them to take control of their skin health and improve their lives in unimaginable ways. My story is a testament to the fact that change is possible. I've healed my skin and no longer suffer from rosacea, wrinkles, dark circles, or any of the issues I struggled with before. I look younger now at forty than I did in my twenties!

Healing my skin was a holistic process, and it started with improving the love I have for myself. The inner healing was the tonic. The more I started to love myself, the more I wanted to nourish and nurture my skin, to show myself the appreciation and tenderness I deserved to feel. Through years of trial and error, I discovered the best skincare tools, including microneedling, which has become the bedrock of my business and my journey to self-love.

INTRODUCTION

This book is a culmination of my life's work and experiences. Through my personal stories, explanations, and practical advice, I hope to help you navigate the world of skincare with confidence and heal the wounds that have likely stayed hidden for most of your life. I hope that you'll find the sacred space within you that speaks and knows the truth, and that you'll come to love yourself—inside and out—without conditions. I hope that you come to know that the power to have beautiful, youthful, glowing skin is in your hands.

If what I've learned about skin and the tools I've developed and share in this book help just one person, I will consider my life well-lived. I hope you are that one.

Scan the QR code below to
access my YouTube channel

CHAPTER 1

BEAUTY & SELF-LOVE

When I think back to my earliest memories of skincare, I realize now that it was my first love. I started working for a cosmetics company when I was fourteen years old, captivated by the promise of each bottle, irresistible to a girl who felt plain and forgettable. I'd walk around my school with the latest AVON catalog, selling makeup and skincare products to make enough money to buy some for myself. I was mesmerized by what appeared to be magic contained in jars: glowing skin, youthfulness, elegance, and femininity.

I was enchanted. I believed there was something in those potions that could fix how I felt about myself. I was awkward in my own skin and longed for the ease and grace of women who looked flawless. They had a confidence that I lacked. I wanted to be beautiful, and it seemed to me that beauty came in bottles.

Beauty meant belonging to a whole world beyond my small Lithuanian village. It meant belonging and acceptance and the courage to be exactly who you wanted to be. Beauty was the highest form of self-expression, and it was achieved through the skin. Beauty hinted at something I couldn't name just yet, something that I believed was lacking in my own life.

While working for AVON, I attended seminars and conferences where I learned about the biology of skin and skincare products and ingredients. But I was only fifteen, still a child with an impressionable mind, desperate to be beautiful and seen. This repeated exposure to the skincare industry and talk of perfect skin led to obsession. I noticed all the ways I didn't meet the beauty standards that were being marketed and sold. I noticed all the flaws in my appearance, painfully aware of my acne and dry, dull skin, my thin lips, my underweight frame—all the differences between me and other women that made me feel average and kept me from feeling beautiful. My teenage world became hyperfocused on the pursuit of perfection. I thought only about skin and appearances, and this became the standard by which—certainly for me—all beauty was measured. It was the start of a chronic cycle of self-doubt and anxiety that would take me more than twenty years to heal.

I wanted the power to erase my perceived defects, to fix what I felt inside. I believed that if I could perfect my skin, I could perfect my life. I imagined a future where clear, glowing skin would open doors for me and create the opportunities I craved. This led me to study to become an esthetician.

Then, in my twenties, I decided to leave Lithuania. I wanted to play a bigger part in the world, to be at the heart of the thrill and adventure beyond the boundaries of what felt like an insignificant life. I wanted style and excitement—I wanted more. I chose Miami because it was a fusion of everything I was looking for: sunny beaches, beautiful people, rich culture, great food. I'm not a materialistic person, but the allure of the city and its luxury was intoxicating. It wasn't so much what people had or didn't have that drew me in; it was the way it all made me feel. Miami and the idea of moving there made me feel like I would finally be *somebody* doing *something*.

And, indeed, Miami still fills me with passion—the glamour, the bold cultures, the vibrant celebration of color and individuality. It's shaped who I am today and surrounds me with endless inspiration. But moving

1. BEAUTY & SELF-LOVE

there came with its challenges, especially for a young woman from a distant country with deep insecurities. Miami is a city of duality—rich, poor, celebrities, and everyday people. It's real, and that's what I appreciate about it. But the city's obsession with "perfection" and the latest plastic surgery trends can create immense pressure to conform. Whatever insecurities I arrived with in my twenties only amplified. I started getting lip and temple fillers to change the shape of my face and Botox to hide my premature aging lines. On top of that, I was broke and working two jobs, Monday to Sunday, just to make ends meet. It was exhausting. The city had won my heart, but the harsh reality of life in a foreign country on my own was taking a toll on me—mentally, emotionally, and physically—especially on my skin.

I hit rock bottom in 2017 when my body finally said no. I was experiencing chronic pain and landed in the emergency room three times in one month. I was sick and unhealthy, but each time I saw a doctor, they couldn't find a cause. I remember telling God that I couldn't live with the pain anymore—the pain in my body and the pain in my soul; that I would rather die than continue to suffer like I was. It was an extremely dark time in my life.

Despite persistent physical symptoms, I was told that it was all in my head and what I needed was therapy. But I'd spent a lifetime building a connection with my body. And even though I had placed my focus on the superficial aspects of my skin, a little voice inside told me something I quietly already knew about myself: that the cost of the way I was living my life, as well as the emotional toll of the loathing I projected onto myself and my skin, had finally rebounded. It was then that I knew that I could not give up until I had my answers. My body was communicating with me, and it was telling me that it was time for change.

I eventually found the holistic doctor who changed my life. He asked me more than two hundred questions during my first consultation, which lasted roughly three hours. He questioned everything, including my lifestyle, diet, how and where I lived, my job, my happiness with myself and others, and my relationships. He ran a battery of tests which revealed that I had mercury toxicity, a yeast infection that had caused symptoms for three years, and several parasites in my body. I was diagnosed with Hashimoto's thyroiditis, leaky gut syndrome, rosacea, and prediabetes. It was a shock, but I was relieved that I finally had answers. I'd finally found the root of my physical symptoms, which allowed me to shift my focus and all of my energy to finding the solutions. I decided that it was time to stop living the toxic life that I was living physically, emotionally, mentally, and spiritually. I was thirty years old.

This was the turning point in my life. Like many people searching for answers, I read books by researchers and healers to better understand my diagnoses and what I could do to heal myself. I stopped drinking alcohol, chose foods that were nourishing, and moved my body in gentler, more loving ways. I started doing regular enemas, meditation, yoga, and therapy. I listened to what my body and my skin were telling me, turning toward what was good and healthy for me.

It wasn't a quick fix. It was slow, often uncomfortable, and extremely vulnerable. But something started to happen when I listened to my body. First, I began to experience a deep compassion for myself. Like so many people, I'd been carrying pain and insecurity with me for years. When I gave myself permission to feel that pain, I loved what I saw. And then, my skin started to heal. After all the years of exploiting it and treating it with such disgust, my skin finally responded to love.

During this time, I stopped doing Botox and fillers because I no longer needed them. Removing alcohol and caffeine from my diet, in addition to doing weekly enemas to clear my gut, completely reversed my rosacea and my prediabetes and my skin started to glow—naturally! The more love I directed toward myself, the healthier my skin became. The love I had for myself expanded, which allowed me to

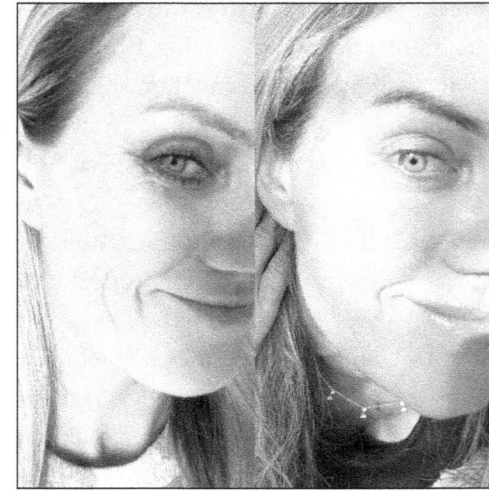

1. BEAUTY & SELF-LOVE

finally realize my purpose: to dedicate my life to helping other women overcome struggles with their own skin and empower them to experience *real* self-love.

When you awaken, everything shifts. You see the world through a different lens. You stop judging yourself and others, and you start living from your heart. Life becomes more about how you can help others and less about what you can gain for yourself. You become more present, more kind, and more aware of the short time you have here on Earth. I realized that my purpose is to share what I've learned on my own journey with my skin. My obsession with skin and skincare throughout the years gave me so much knowledge and insight that I built a multimillion-dollar skincare brand that has helped thousands of women all over the world overcome their own struggles with their skin.

Good skincare is not a luxury—it's an act of self-love. Taking time to cleanse, hydrate, and protect your skin is a way to honor your body. But no serum or cream can replace the soothing effect of radiance that comes from within. True self-love goes beyond the surface; it's about embracing authentic living and enhancing the power of your natural beauty. This philosophy eventually led me to create tools and products that reflect my belief in the skin's ability to heal itself.

I'm at a wonderful point in my life. I wrote this book, run a successful company, and have a family. All of my hard work and perseverance has paid off, and I can hardly believe I've created this life for myself. Reflecting on how far I've come, I'm struck by this powerful truth: Desperation, although it feels unbearable in the moment, can be an incredible catalyst for change. Desperation really *is* a gift. It's those moments of rock bottom, those dark nights of the soul, those times when you thought you've been beaten by life that allow you to let go of everything you're not and finally open yourself to everything you have the potential to be.

The same is true for your skin. What probably brought you to this book is desperation: the desperation of thousands of dollars spent on products and tools only to see no change in your skin; the desperation of the grief you feel at the loss of control over your skin; the desperation you feel when you reflect on the years you've spent trying to conceal or diminish the truth of who you are because you're afraid you're not enough. Whatever desperation brought you here, I see you. It's time to let go of the pressure you've put on your skin to look a certain way and respect its natural rhythms. What you needed all along was to listen more intently to the ancient wisdom of the skin.

I recommend that you read *Gut and Psychology Syndrome*[1] by Dr. Natasha Campbell-McBride, who uses a nutritional approach as a treatment. She is recognized as one of the world's leading experts in treating children and adults with learning disabilities and other mental disorders, as well as children and adults with digestive and immune disorders. Her books have also helped in the treatment of ADHD, autism, depression, and schizophrenia.

From Insecure to Self-loving Divine Woman

For centuries, women have been told that beauty is power. Historically, they were rarely given a seat at any table of significance, so most of them were left with their only permissible power: the power of being attractive. Ancient cultures celebrated the physical characteristics of women; at times when they had limited access to education, professions, and autonomy, beauty was their key to having control over their own life.[2] Ironically, possessing beauty didn't really give women the freedom and power they were looking for—rather, beauty standards continue to oppress women, reinforcing their dependency on external validation.

Skin, particularly, was prized as the highest form of beauty. Fair, unblemished skin was considered a sign of wealth and privilege because it meant that you weren't spending your days working outdoors in the sun, but had the luxury of staying inside.[3] Unblemished skin was a sign of social

---

1. Campbell-MBride, N. (2015). *Gut and Psychology Syndrome: Natural Treatment for Autism, Dyspraxia, A.D.D., Dyslexia, A.D.H.D., Depression, Schizophrenia*. Medinform.
2. Wolf, N. (1991). *The Beauty Myth: How Images of Beauty Are Used Against Women*. HarperCollins.
3. Goodman, R. M. (2019). *The History of Makeup and Skin Care: Beauty Through the Ages*. Routledge.

1. BEAUTY & SELF-LOVE

status. Women in ancient cultures went to extreme lengths to lighten their skin, including using toxic lead-based powders. I don't think much has changed. Despite the research that continues to highlight the toxicity of many skincare ingredients and the risks involved with skin augmentation procedures, the yearning for desirable skin persists—no matter the cost.

Although women now have greater access to education, careers, and leadership than at any other point in history, the heritage of beauty as power continues to shape modern society. Social media has created a culture of comparison that defines today's beauty standards of femininity and womanhood and discards the multifaceted characteristics that make up a woman's identity—her intelligence, her innovativeness, her uniqueness. If women continue to hold themselves to impossible beauty standards— standards that keep them uncomfortable in their own skin—they will deprive themselves of their true power: the Divine Woman.

The Divine Woman is your most authentic self; it nurtures you from a place of intention and self-love rather than a place of criticism and perfectionism. The Divine Woman is balanced. She knows your strengths and your weaknesses, and she accepts them all as you—*without judgment, without pressure, without condition*. The Divine Woman reclaims the parts of yourself that you've hidden out of shame and fear. By re-examining your own personal beauty beliefs, you'll start to reclaim the Divine Woman in you. She understands that true beauty is a personal and divine expression of everything that you are. The Divine Woman embodies a deeper connection with yourself and your skin.

In my own journey, it was only once I shifted away from the demands of the world outside of me and connected with the longings of the voice within that I unlocked the healing power of my own skin. I needed to open myself up to a more inclusive definition of beauty and find the self-love that I had denied for so long. It was only from this place that I was able to connect with my Divine Woman, and it's only from her that I'm able to connect with you. She's my most authentic, intelligent, and creative self. She has deep reverence for the skin I'm in, and from here, I'm able to pour into myself and into all the women I help.

Self-love is the beginning of becoming a Divine Woman. This journey starts with realizing the ways you've internalized these restrictive skin beauty standards. In the pursuit for flawless skin, perhaps you didn't realize that what keeps your skin sick is likely coming from within. Toxicity doesn't only enter your body from harmful external environments. Sometimes the toxicity that is keeping your skin from healing is the way you feel about yourself. Your body is the environment your skin exists in, and taking care of it means healing the relationship you have with it. The language of self-love means not *fixing* your skin but *honoring* it. Through years of working with hundreds of women and reflecting on my own journey, I've found that when a woman is able to make that mental shift, she starts to embody her divinity.

Before I discovered my divinity, I, like so many of you, tried everything I possibly could externally to change the way I looked. Maybe you've been there too—spending money you don't have chasing a perception of beauty you've idealized only to realize that each adjustment highlights further imperfections, feeding a cycle of self-disapproval.

Even after hitting rock bottom, my insecurities didn't automatically disappear. When I first started posting videos on YouTube, sharing the journey I was on with my skin, I was met with criticism and ridicule for everything from my accent to my appearance despite my age. If you've ever dared to be vulnerable while still on the journey of learning to love yourself, you'll know how exposed and sensitive you can feel in that space. Even though I was coming to understand that I'm a woman of worth no matter what other people say, I'd spent so much of my life building an identity around my appearance and the approval of others that it took time to separate myself from external opinions and trust what I knew to be true. I, like so many other women, still have to remind myself where my real value lies from time to time. Through extensive research, hard work, and personal experience, I built a skincare brand from the ground up and am now considered a master in microneedling, helping clients from all over the world heal their skin and their relationship with themselves. But, some days, I still feel like the girl from my small village. Can you relate?

1. BEAUTY & SELF-LOVE

The truth is, insecurities are a part of the human experience. Some may never disappear completely, but they don't need to control your life. Most women experience some level of insecurity about aging because, in most societies, aging has been connected to a loss of value. Many women fear this loss of control over their place in society and even fear for the safety and security of their relationships. The double standard that exists for men and women in society has created an enormous amount of pressure for women to be perfect and to avoid aging at all costs. Wrinkles, pigmentation, dark circles under the eyes, broken blood vessels, and dry skin are all common as you get older, yet you're left with very few examples of real women to show you how to deal with these skin issues in ways that don't include extreme courses of action.

This is why I do what I do. I want to normalize aging skin and empower you to treat your skin with the respect that it deserves while you give it what it needs. There is a simple way to unlock the wisdom of your own skin, to use the medicine of the body to protect and preserve this remarkable organ. You have the power to change your skin story, to change the story you're telling yourself about who you are and why you matter. You have the power to write the story of the rest of your life. You don't need to wait for skin perfection before you start listening to the Divine Woman within you. I didn't. This is how you change the world—and heal your skin.

The Awareness That You Have the Power to Change

Your skin has an incredible ability to heal and change. The same can be said for you. Despite the challenges you have likely faced in your life, you're here today, in this moment, present and alive to your life. When I talk about holistic skincare, I'm talking about this too: your resilience, your ability to heal, your potential to transform your life. Holistic skin starts and ends with your power to change.

The journey from insecurity to self-love brings forth a revelation: If you're no longer bound by the limitations of society's beauty standards, you're opening yourself up to your Divine Woman and listening for her voice when insecurities abound. You're connecting with your skin and creating rituals that ground you in your own body, and you're at long last accessing your power. You're no longer a passive recipient of your life; you are an active contributor to your personal story.

Awareness is the foundation for change. The fact that you're here now means that awareness has crept into your consciousness. You're becoming aware of all the ways you're sabotaging your skin, of all the self-destructive patterns that keep your skin sick. You're becoming aware that it's time to take ownership of your skin and that you already have everything you need to do so. Your curiosity has brought you here—and it's curiosity that brings you to the answers. In a world where you have little control over what happens, you're becoming aware that you *can* control the decisions you make about your health, your skin, and your relationship with yourself.

When you approach skincare with awareness, you learn to listen to your skin. You recognize its signals, understand how to meet its needs, and tend to it with compassion. This connection fosters a deep sense of self-acceptance. You're no longer trying to fix your skin because you disapprove of it, you're nurturing it as an extension of your divinity.

The Divine Woman, one who understands her power, finds simple pleasure in washing her face because it's an act of cleansing after a day of showing her face to the world. A sacred ritual is created when you take the time to feel the skin beneath your fingers when cleansing it. It's a radical act of self-love to touch yourself with such intentionality, a radical act of defiance in today's fast-paced world to slow down and spend this time with your skin. Whenever you take the time to dedicate this attention to yourself, you're honoring the divine in you and creating a mindful approach to caring for your skin. Many women have forgotten the simple act of caring for themselves in this way. In the rush of modern living, your skincare may be at the bottom of your list of to-dos. But this is where sincere self-love starts. If you don't believe you are worth taking a few minutes in the evening to cleanse your face, how can you possibly show up face-first in other areas of your life?

Mindful skincare rituals are framed by mindful practices that offer a complete view of you as a human being. This means practices like meditation and journaling are good for your skin too! Taking time to meditate on your skin and focusing on what you would like to heal is a powerful practice. Visualize your skin the way you want to see it. See yourself as the confident person you're becoming, free from skin insecurities. Journal about the habits in your life that might be holding you back. Have you noticed certain responses from your skin when you eat particular foods? How does your skin react to caffeine? Is your skin thirsty? Are you sleeping well at night? These are all important questions to explore when journaling. Likewise, consider the ingredients in your skincare products and whether they're helping or hindering your skin health. Is your skin trying to communicate with you every time you use certain products? As a Divine Woman, you'll want to align your skincare products with your values, so asking yourself if products and ingredients are in your skin's and the environment's best interest is a key consideration for holistic skincare.

This journey to authentically connecting with yourself requires tapping into the persistence and bravery that come from your spiritual connection to the divine. This divine strength offers you the power to persist, even if things take time. It's the courage to be disliked when you bring countercultural wisdom forward. It's the strength to stand up for what's right in the face of strong opposition, even if that means saying no to popular skincare trends and trusting your own body. It's daring to go bare-faced into the world, with nothing to hide behind, and affirming your belief in yourself just as you are.

These small acts of self-love might seem insignificant at first, but they build confidence over time. Each time you do something kind for yourself, each time you make decisions that nurture your skin, you're telling yourself and your skin that you love it. You're creating a positive feedback loop because instead of waiting to feel love for your skin—instead of waiting for perfection—you're showing your skin love right now and reinforcing the belief that your skin is enough just as it is. This practice creates more positive feelings, which increases the chances of you repeating them! This is how small acts bring about large changes; this is how a decision as simple as making time to cleanse your face each night leads to transformation.

Somewhere along the road you chose. You chose the story you wanted your life to tell, you chose to spend time taking care of your skin, you chose to be intentional about the nourishment you put into your body and on your skin. You chose. This is how you change the way you feel about yourself. This is how you renew your relationship with your skin. You choose.

Defining Beauty Holistically

The demands and stress of the modern world and the staggering amount of misinformation regarding beauty and self-care that the average woman encounters on a daily basis means that many women have lost touch with how to nourish not only their skin but themselves. Holistic beauty has emerged as a response to this disconnection. Its practices are rooted in getting in touch with the parts of yourself that respect and reflect balance and a state of well-being. Holistic beauty invites you to reconnect with your skin and skincare routine in meaningful ways. If you let it, your skin can open you up to deeper self-healing practices, letting go of the chase for perfection and nurturing yourself physically, emotionally, mentally, and spiritually.

Holistic beauty is harmony between skin and soul. Where there's dysregulation, there's likely a detachment from self. Where you find yourself in your life right now might look something like dysregulation—a dysregulated nervous system as a result of trauma and disconnection from people you love because you're ashamed to show up in your skin. What so often gets overlooked when dealing with the results of trauma and stress on the body is taking a trauma-informed approach to skincare as well. What's often not said out loud can be written across your skin.

Holistic skincare considers that your skin is a part of a larger biological system: your entire body. It doesn't exist in isolation from everything else that happens anatomically. Your skin will react to trauma and stress in the same way the rest of your body does: with inflammation. Inflammation is an essential response from your immune system to defend against infection and damage; in other words, it's your body's way of protecting and healing. But stressors or trauma can disrupt the natural order of your biological system, and often this inflammatory response reverberates the loudest across your skin. So understanding the relationship between your emotions, experiences, mental state, and skin is vital for establishing holistic beauty and skincare practices.

Trauma is experienced differently by different people. Many women disregard their own traumatic experiences because they minimize the psychological and emotional impact of those experiences. Women have been socialized to absorb all of their anger and not express it, and they're rewarded by society, particularly men, when they're submissive and easy to be around. As a result, they often betray themselves by denying the effects of their experiences. They put everyone else first and consider their needs last, if at all. What they get as a result is usually a deeply troubled subconscious and a body and skin that are saying all the things they can't.

Emotional pain leaves scars. No matter the type of pain or the severity, it will find a way to be felt. It may take years, decades, or even lifetimes, but it will demand to be felt. That demand can manifest as tension, inflammation, illness, or skin disorders. The more you try to suppress this pain, the more trauma you inflict on your body, mind, and skin. It's a vicious cycle. If what brought you to this book is a disordered relationship with your skin and chronic skin issues that you haven't been able to heal, then I hope that you'll trust me when I ask you to start *here*. To start the healing here, right where you are: soul healing. Soul healing must be your companion on this road.

Earlier I discussed that the Divine Woman is in touch with her most authentic self, but soul healing starts when you ask yourself what some of the blockages are that keep you from connecting with your authenticity. What emotional pain are you carrying that could be causing you and your skin to suffer? What trauma wounds are you holding? What fears have numbed you? These emotions are powerful triggers in your body's system, and developing self-love means giving yourself permission to finally feel them. Holistic beauty includes the beauty that radiates from within from genuine love for every part of you. It means finally being present in your body, in your skin. Presence that allows you to listen and restore your body's natural systems of healing and rejuvenation.

Now that you're starting to see yourself as a whole being and starting to see every part of your design as interconnected and communicating, which parts of yourself and your story have you silenced over the years because of the fear of what lies there? It's time to give yourself a voice and listen to what's going on inside you. The trauma you're hiding from is distorting your view of yourself, and it's impossible to develop self-love and heal when you don't know who you need to love. The parts of you that you most fear are the parts of you that will heal your skin. This is how you practice holistic skincare.

This journey is going to require that you carve out sacred spaces for your healing. If you want to heal your skin, if you want to glow, if you're searching for beauty, transcend the perceived limitations of your skin and start to care for yourself—mind, body, and soul. Skincare products and tools are only one facet of holistic beauty. Holistic beauty understands that these aid in the healing of your skin, but alone they aren't the cure. Honoring yourself as a Divine Woman means taking one step at a time and rising up to meet your needs. That small step will look different for each person. It could mean therapy for emotional wounds that you still carry, choosing foods that support and strengthen every cell in your body, drinking more water and making the time to get better sleep, meditating and communing with nature, grounding your body and soul at the foot of big trees and skies. Healing isn't about overwhelming yourself with more unachievable goals; it's about recognizing that these are holistic skincare practices. These are beauty tools too.

CHAPTER 2

UNDERSTANDING SKINCARE BASICS

The Science Behind Skincare

By now, it should be clear that skincare is about more than just your daily routine. It's a reflection of the kind of respect and consideration you give to yourself as a person—mind, body, and soul. When you approach your skincare holistically, you go beyond superficial treatments and putting bandaids on symptoms, instead embracing a deeper connection with your body and your humanity through self-love. But self-love isn't just about the way you feel about yourself; it's also about knowledge—knowing what your skin needs and why. Effective skincare starts with understanding the biology of your skin and the science behind how it functions.

But let's be honest: Skincare science can feel overwhelming. Not everyone has the knowledge of an esthetician or dermatologist, and for some, all the talk of ingredients, layers, and functions might seem unnecessary. Perhaps it seems easier for you to trust the brands you've trusted all your life or the routine you've followed for years. And that's okay. But here's something I want you to know: While the science of skin might be intimidating, understanding it, even on a basic level, will empower you to make informed choices and foster a more loving relationship with your skin. Holistic skincare isn't just about vanity; it's about wellness and looking after yourself in a way that goes beyond surface beauty and toward addressing the root causes of issues while maintaining the wholeness of your entire body.

Your skin is a vital organ, and it does far more than just hold everything together. It's your first line of defense against the world: pollution, harmful bacteria, toxins, and the sun's damaging rays. It even regulates your body's temperature and communicates emotions. Think of blushing when you feel shy! When you consider what it means to care for your skin, it shouldn't feel like a luxury you can't afford, but a way of looking after and protecting one of the most important parts of your body.

Simply put, at the heart of skincare science lies the support you can give to this vital protective barrier. When this barrier is strong, your body is well defended against environmental stressors. This is easy to spot because a strong skin barrier means smooth, radiant skin, like when you wake up from deep, restful sleep! But a compromised skin barrier—caused by harsh skincare ingredients, overexposure to sunlight without protection, inadequate hydration, a lack of restorative sleep or a nourishing diet—can leave you open to vulnerabilities like dryness, redness, wrinkles, and dark spots.

I once had a client who did all the worst things possible for her skin. She didn't wear sunscreen, smoked cigarettes and drank alcohol, didn't get enough sleep, overdid exfoliation and actives, ate lots of sugary treats, and overall was very hard on herself. When she finally accepted that the causes of her premature aging were these bad habits, she reached out for a simple skincare plan starting with my dermarollers, peptides, sunscreen, vitamin C repair cream, and sheet masks; she also let go of her bad habits. After only eleven months, her skin had visibly improved; she had fewer wrinkles and was practically glowing. A lot of my clients' stories are like this. It takes good habits and good skincare.

Think of your skin as your built-in armor that absorbs and deflects punches from the environment, shielding you from physical harm. And the best part? Your skin already knows how to do all of this on its own. The only science

2. UNDERSTANDING SKINCARE BASICS

that matters is understanding how to support it using a few simple routines and practices that optimize its natural cycles.

Outdated Skincare Beliefs

Now that you have a very basic understanding—and likely appreciation—for the science of skin and its care, you're probably asking yourself, "If skincare is so simple, why does it feel so complicated?" The truth is, so much of what you've been told and taught about skincare isn't founded on science or evidence, but rather anecdotal outdated beliefs, deceiving marketing tactics, and skincare myths that have been passed down through generations. These ideas have been repeated so often they sound like facts. In many ways, skincare for most women isn't just a routine—it's a legacy.

As a young girl, part of your development included absorbing—likely without critical evaluation—the beliefs of the women around you. Part of the socialization process of human development includes your ability to learn what to do and what not to do to become a functioning member of society. This process is not limited to social behavior; your brain is wired to soak up all the information around you and draw conclusions about the world based on what you learn, including beauty routines and how to care for your skin. These beliefs persist not necessarily because they're true, but because they're familiar, and when something feels familiar, you're unlikely to stop and ask yourself, "Is this even good for my skin?"

Early on in my skincare journey, a friend recommended that I skip my morning face wash to help with my acne. I was completely skeptical. How could *less* cleansing be better? But after years of battling with my skin, I was willing to try anything. To my surprise, my skin actually improved! And the science of skin health backs this up. Dermatologists now suggest that cleansing more than once a day strips your skin of its natural oils, causing it to produce more oils to achieve balance. Your morning cleanse also disrupts the millions of bacteria and microorganisms that call your skin home and do some of their most important work at night—creating microbiomes that protect your skin from harmful bacteria, environmental stressors, and inflammation. Between the time you go to bed and the time you wake up, it's unlikely that your skin has been exposed to dirt and grime, so by skipping your morning face wash, you honor the essential ecosystem of your skin by allowing the natural oils and microbiome to do their jobs. This results in clear, glowy skin, fewer wrinkles, balanced sebum (oil) production—which means no more pimples, blackheads, whiteheads, and clogged pores—reduced skin sensitivity, improved hydration, and a stronger, healthier skin barrier.

Yet, despite the science, outdated skincare beliefs persist, and it's not hard to see why. For decades, women have been the focus of skincare marketing campaigns, bombarded with messages that to achieve flawless, younger skin, they only need to buy more products. I know this because I fell for it too. I fell for every trend and product that claimed it would cure my skin concerns and make me look and feel better. Looking back, I realize that the marketing tactic of these big companies was to prey on my insecurities rather than genuinely help my skin.

The beauty industry, worth $677 billion, makes its bottom line by selling the idea that more is better, and that your skin is a problem to be solved rather than an organ to be cared for. When this is the narrative, it's easy to feel like you're *not doing enough*, and this can be exhausting. These feelings are completely valid. Large beauty corporations aren't selling skincare; they're selling a lifetime buy-in to their products because they're offering perfection and eternal youthfulness. Both are an invention of their industry.

Their strategy isn't a solution; it's selling you a problem you didn't even know you had. And this isn't your fault. The beauty industry has spent decades selling women the recommendation that they need to meet certain narrow beauty standards in order to be accepted, valued, and loved. These are the basic needs of all human beings, and the industry exploits these by offering you a false sense of control, hope, and belonging, all of which will be earned if you buy their product and achieve flawless skin. Or so they say. When you feel insecure or empty inside, you become more receptive to the influence of this messaging. As long as skincare beliefs are determined by the industries that thrive on profit from your pain, they'll continue to push outdated beliefs. It's no wonder you feel so overwhelmed and dissatisfied.

2. UNDERSTANDING SKINCARE BASICS

Not All Natural Ingredients Are Created Equal

When discussing skincare ingredients, it's important to recognize that natural (i.e., from plant sources) does not always mean safe or nonirritating, and synthetic does not automatically mean harmful or toxic. Understanding why and how the beauty industry sets and maintains outdated skincare beliefs, it's easy to see why, recently, consumers—now better informed about the products they use and the potential harm and benefits thereof—are searching for safer, nontoxic alternatives. They want good-for-you ingredients that are free from harmful substances like fragrance, parabens, gluten, sodium lauryl sulphate, and more, while still living up to their claims and producing results.

This has led to a demand for "clean" products—those that aren't harmful to your health or the health of the planet. However, with this rise in consumer awareness and demand from the public for more transparency from the beauty industry, the word "natural" has become a seductive marketing tool, with big companies taking advantage of consumers' desires to make more sustainable and healthier choices. This has led to a rise in what's been termed *greenwashing*—the advertising promise of products, including skincare products, as being more sustainable and cleaner than they really are.

And the problem starts at the very top of the beauty chain. There are no clear regulations on what "natural" actually means in beauty products, and there's a deafening silence from the industry regarding information for consumers to help educate them on whether all ingredients derived from plant sources are actually safer than synthetic ingredients, and whether all synthetic ingredients are harmful. For example, certain mushrooms found in nature are organic and natural but can be deadly if consumed. Similarly, many natural ingredients in skincare can be highly irritating. Essential oils, for instance, are completely natural, yet excessive use can cause severe skin irritation, redness, or even burns.

Another good example is vitamin C. The purest and most natural form is ascorbic acid, but applying lemon or lime juice directly to the skin can severely damage the skin's protective barrier. So, while an ingredient may be natural, its concentration and application method determine its safety and effectiveness.

It's also important to mention that natural ingredients seldom undergo the same thorough testing as synthetic ones. Why would they when they're natural, right? Synthetic, man-made components are usually produced in controlled settings with exact combinations that have been checked for safety and efficacy, while natural ingredients may exhibit different levels of concentration and effectiveness due to variations in harvesting and processing methods, resulting in varying outcomes—not all of them being safe. For example, one bottle of tea-tree oil may have a different concentration than another, which can impact how safe and effective it is despite its antibacterial properties.

My goal in skincare formulation is always to create products that are gentle, effective, nonirritating, and toxic-free. My aim is to use natural ingredients whenever possible, but all the products in my Gin Amber Beauty range are certified ToxicFree® (by the ToxicFree Foundation) and are highly effective, sustainable ingredients in safe concentrations and forms. My team at Gin Amber Beauty is committed to research and development that meets the highest standards and prioritizes the health and satisfaction of all of our clients. This means the strictest regulations for all our ingredients that have been proven, with science, to be good for you and your skin.

In many cases, synthetic ingredients are carefully designed to stabilize formulas, reduce irritation, and enhance performance. In short, a well-balanced formulation can require synthetic components to ensure safety, stability, and effectiveness.

So, the next time you're tempted by the natural skincare aisle, take a moment to look at what's actually in the product. Look at the label, the parent company, and each ingredient's reason for being there. Don't underestimate your power and freedom to make choices that are good for you and your skin. Understand your own skin's needs, and don't be afraid to mix natural ingredients with well-formulated synthetic ones. After all,

2. UNDERSTANDING SKINCARE BASICS

the goal is holistically healthy, glowing skin, and sometimes that means combining the best of both worlds.

Skincare Myths and Truths

By now I hope you have a better understanding of your skin's health and how misconceptions and misleading advertising have shaped a great deal of the collective skincare beliefs. Modern research has debunked many of the myths that have been passed down through generations regarding how to care for skin. Now, with a deeper understanding of dermatology and greater access to evidence-based truths, it is essential to modernize not only skincare rituals but also skincare knowledge in order to embrace holistic beauty.

Below is a list of common skincare myths and their truths. Reviewing these will allow you to evaluate the ways you currently care for your skin and empower you to make science-backed changes if need be.

MYTH	TRUTH
The more you exfoliate your skin, the better.	Over-exfoliating can damage your skin by stripping away its natural oils and disrupting the skin barrier. Limit exfoliation to once a week.
Oily skin doesn't need moisturizer.	All skin types, including oily skin, benefit from moisturizer. Skipping moisturizer can actually cause your skin to produce more oil to compensate for dryness, leading to breakouts.
Pores can open and close.	Pores are tiny openings in your skin that allow oil and sweat to reach the surface, but they do not have muscles to open and close like doors. When they are clogged with dirt or oil, they can appear larger because they are more visible. When skin is hydrated, it appears more smooth, giving the appearance of smaller pores. Heat or steam can temporarily soften dirt, oil, or dead skin cells in your pores, making them easier to clean and, therefore, appear smaller, but they don't physically change size.

MYTH	TRUTH
Sunscreen is only needed on sunny days.	UV rays are present year round and can penetrate clouds and windows. Daily sunscreen use, regardless of weather, is essential for protecting against premature aging and skin cancer. I only recommend mineral-based, toxic-free sunscreen. Chemical sunscreens contain toxic ingredients that are absorbed into the body and can disrupt hormone systems, and have even been found in breastmilk and to cross the blood-brain barrier.
Skincare products need to tingle or burn to work.	Sensations like tingling or burning can actually indicate irritation, especially for sensitive skin. While some products may cause slight discomfort, this is not a prerequisite to garner results.
Acne is caused by dirty skin.	Acne is primarily influenced by gut health—what you eat, environmental stressors, hormones, genetics, and bacteria. While cleansing is important, over-washing or harsh scrubbing can exacerbate acne by irritating your skin and disrupting its natural balance, leading to higher production of oils and clogged pores.
Higher SPF (sun protection factor) offers better protection.	SPF measures how long you can stay in the sun without burning, but a higher SPF does not mean stronger protection. For example, SPF 25 blocks 96 percent of UVB rays, while SPF 50 blocks 98 percent, making the difference minimal. SPF mainly protects against sunburn-causing UVB rays but does not measure protection against UVA rays, which contribute to aging and skin damage. A higher SPF also creates a false sense of security which leads people into staying out in the sun longer and skipping reapplication, overexposing themselves to the harmful UV rays. Additionally, the ratio of UVA protection decreases as the SPF number increases. This leads to higher risk of skin cancer, exposure to free radicals, and a weaker immunity system. To ensure you're getting equal protection, make sure to look for broad spectrum sunscreens.

2. UNDERSTANDING SKINCARE BASICS

MYTH	TRUTH
Dermarollers cause scarring. / You can't use dermarollers at home.	Dermarolling is a form of microneedling that involves the use of a handheld tool that is rolled across your skin to form micropunctures that stimulate collagen production. Many dermatologists discourage dermarolling at home because 99 percent of dermarollers on the market are fake. These fake tools use cheap metal wheels instead of individual needles, grating your skin, damaging skin cells, and causing scarring. Proper dermarollers have individual needles that penetrate your skin independently, meaning they're not dragged across your skin. Gin Amber Beauty CE medical-certified Real Individual Needles® dermarollers are 100 percent safe to use at home and do not cause scarring. Proper dermarolling stimulates collagen, elastin, and keratin production in your skin and improves product absorption. Dermarolling is safe for most people but should be avoided on active acne, open wounds, raised scars, psoriasis, fungal infections, skin cancer, moles, and warts.
You must bleed in order to see results from skin procedures.	Bleeding is not necessary to see results from treatments like dermarolling. Some professional treatments may involve deeper penetration that could cause pinpoint bleeding, especially for acne scars or deep wrinkles. However, not bleeding from a skin procedure should not be taken as a sign that the treatment is not working.
You can't mix retinol and vitamin C.	Both retinol and vitamin C are potent ingredients, but they have different pH levels at which they are most effective. Some dermatologists suggest using them at different times of the day—vitamin C in the morning for its antioxidant benefits and retinol at night for its regenerative properties. However, modern formulations and certain stabilized forms of these ingredients can be combined without causing irritation, depending on your skin's tolerance. The key is to introduce them slowly and monitor your skin's response.

MYTH	TRUTH
Parabens are safe.	Parabens are widely used preservatives in skincare products. Recent studies[4] indicate that parabens act as endocrine disruptors, meaning they interfere with your hormone production, which can lead to fertility issues and breast cancer, as well as high blood pressure.
You can't use actives every day.	Actives are skincare ingredients that target specific skin concerns and can be used daily, depending on the specific ingredient and your skin's tolerance. Actives like vitamin C, hyaluronic acid, and niacinamide are generally safe for everyday use in lower concentrations. Stronger actives like retinoids, AHAs (alpha hydroxy acids), and BHAs (beta hydroxy acids) can cause irritation, sensitivity, or peeling if overused and should be introduced to your skincare routine slowly to monitor your skin's response.
Toners are an essential part of any skincare routine.	Toners were initially developed to remove excess makeup and dirt leftover after cleansing, but modern cleansers have been formulated to cleanse more effectively, eliminating the need for additional steps for thorough cleaning. Additionally, toners, especially alcohol-based toners, can dry out your skin, leading to skin issues you maybe didn't have before you started using them.

---

4. Alnuqaydan A. M. (2024). "The dark side of beauty: an in-depth analysis of the health hazards and toxicological impact of synthetic cosmetics and personal care products." *Frontiers in Public Health*, 12:1439027. doi: 10.3389/fpubh.2024.1439027

CHAPTER 3

THE PSYCHOLOGY OF BEAUTY

Defining Beauty

Do you remember the first time you considered what it meant to be beautiful? Pause here for a moment. Where did this definition of beauty come from? Was it something that was said to you, either about you or about someone else? How did this experience make you feel? Whether you are aware of it or not, this was an important moment in your life; it was the *before* and the *after*. Before you were aware of the silent rules of beauty that exist and persist in the world around you, and after you realized the power these rules had to influence the way you see yourself and others.

As a woman, it's likely that beauty is not something you discovered on your own; it's something you were taught. Moments such as the one you just reflected on are potent experiences that conditioned you into believing what is considered to be desirable and what is not. Observing the way other women showed up in the world, as well as the way these women were accepted or rejected, you absorbed rules about what should be visible and what should be hidden. For many, this was a painful realization. Being held to beauty standards that were exclusive by nature meant a lifetime of being overlooked, and trying—and failing—to measure up.

This is the psychology of beauty, a critique of the complexities that live beneath the surface of your life—and your skin. The psychology of beauty aims to unravel why and how some women feel the way they do about the way that they look, and, most importantly, to hold a safe, compassionate space for women to explore the impact that beauty propaganda, including unattainable skin ideals, has had on their self-esteem.

It's not easy to be a woman in the world. Despite your remarkable ability to adapt to the demands placed on you by society, this resilience, in my experience, comes with a cost. You're burned out from the pursuit of perfection, stressed about the money it costs to use the right products to hold onto youth, and all the while aware of the reality that society only values you for a short time before it moves on to *younger, better, more beautiful*. The pressure of holding all of this tension in your body, mind, and soul is deeply detrimental to your mental and physical well-being.

But seeking approval from society is not a failing on the part of women; it's not vanity or pride. Healing this part of yourself is not as simple as waking up and choosing not to care. Gaining societal approval is a deeply-rooted characteristic of human behavior that is entrenched in the evolutionary need for belonging and acceptance, both of which provide psychological safety. Without these, you feel incredibly vulnerable and exposed, leading to lowered self-esteem, increased anxiety, and overall feelings of worthlessness.

So what does all of this mean? It means it's not your fault that external beauty traits are important to you and that they affect the way you feel about yourself. Research suggests that people with a heightened need for social approval and low self-esteem are at greater risk of depression.[5] Essentially, being a woman in the world puts you at greater risk for mental health struggles when your worth is dependent on the opinions of others.

---

5. Canli, D., & Karaşar, B. (2021). "Predictors of major depressive disorder: The need for social approval and self-esteem." *Alpha Psychiatry*, 22(1), 38–42. doi: 10.5455/apd.97683

3. THE PSYCHOLOGY OF BEAUTY

Social media and culture have further magnified the need for validation. But are you really looking for truth in likes? Or are you chasing something else? The psychology of beauty has a more insightful answer.

The pressure to conform to beauty ideals isn't about looking good. It's about being seen, validated, and respected. Changing the definition of beauty to encompass inner attributes like kindness, intelligence, humor, and resilience is then not only beneficial but necessary. Beauty shouldn't be about the way you look; it should be about the way you live. What if instead of valuing yourself on the smoothness of your skin, you started valuing yourself on the strength you've shown through your most difficult days? Would you see yourself differently then?

Beauty is not about what you *see*, it's about what you *feel*. Your perceptions of beauty are intricately connected to your emotions and experiences. Research shows that attraction isn't solely determined by physical symmetry or how close you come to societal beauty standards; rather, people were considered *more* physically beautiful when they showed traits such as empathy, kindness, and generosity—more so than clear skin.[6]

The way you feel in your skin influences every decision you make, so what if you decided to do something radical and see beauty differently? What if you started caring for your skin from a place of inner strength rather from a place of outer scrutiny? Your definition of beauty is not something that has been handed down to you. It's yours to decide. Holistic skincare is not about going to extreme lengths to be accepted by society; it's about going within to be accepted by yourself.

The Shifting Face of Beauty

Beauty has always been a reflection of its time, influenced by the cultural values and social dynamics of an era. What is considered beautiful today might have been seen as ordinary or even unattractive a hundred years ago, and what was celebrated as beautiful in the past might be considered

---

6. Kononov, N., & Kogut, T. (2024). "Prosocial behaviour enhances evaluation of physical beauty." *British Journal of Social Psychology*, 63(3), 672–89. doi.org/10.1111/bjso.12800

outdated by today's beauty standards. The nature of beauty shows that, in many ways, it's a lot like fashion—constantly evolving, influenced by cultural shifts, societal changes, and the icons who define the look of their time.

Think back to the 1920s, a decade defined by liberation and rebellion against traditional norms. These women rejected not just the restrictive corsets women wore at the time, but the restriction of freedom, using their beauty to claim space and scandalize.

This was a time when women were pushing boundaries, not just socially but aesthetically. They took to embracing a look that was bold, daring, and modern. The beauty trend wasn't just about looking good; it was a statement of independence and defiance. Beauty became a form of rebellion.

But by the '50s, beauty trends again started to shift. The new ideal moved away from the rebellion against gender norms experienced in the Flapper era and settled on a more traditionally feminine ideal, with Marilyn Monroe and Audrey Hepburn at the forefront of '50s culture. Their voluptuous and glamorous nature was capitalized on by the media of the time to remind women that to be desirable and accepted, they needed to fit these feminine molds.

By the '60s and '70s, Twiggy emerged as the face of new femininity during a period of cultural revolution, reflecting a new desire for freedom and self-expression. Her androgynous frame and doll-like eyes embodied the shifting gender norms of the time, embracing individuality and rejecting conformity. In the '80s, Madonna made it clear to women that they could reinvent themselves and not apologize for it. She showed that beauty was not a static concept, but a canvas for personal expression. The '80s were about making a statement, and the beauty trends of the time reflected a culture that was bold, ambitious, and unapologetically larger than life.

Through the '90s and 2000s, minimalism and effortlessness became the hallmark of every Kate Moss adorer, and the internet ushered in an entirely new era. Where for decades beauty ideals had been dictated by Hollywood, the power suddenly moved to the hands of influencers and filters, and now what is deemed beautiful changes more rapidly than ever. But what stands out across decades of beauty history is this: Beauty is not a fixed point on the timeline of humanity. It bends with culture and media, and women get caught in its ebb and flow. It's impossible for women to orient themselves in a constantly changing tide of trends; going to extreme—and sometimes dangerous—lengths to fit whatever construct of femininity society worships at the time.

It's easy to see the kind of pressure that women experience to conform to powerful forces beyond their control time and time again. Beauty changes from decade to decade, leaving women with the lasting effects of their natural selves just never quite being *enough*. I remember feeling like I needed to reinvent myself every few years to keep up. One year it was tanned skin and pin-straight hair; the next it was soft waves and a no-makeup look. I never asked myself what I liked because I was too busy trying to belong.

The compulsion to continually reinvent yourself to find belonging and acceptance in society is consuming women, leaving them with very little time or energy to focus on other areas of their lives. Societies that place value on women only for their appearances continue to preserve cycles of marginalization and sexism. Women internalize these rules—knowingly or unknowingly—and disempower themselves. And the tragedy in all of this is that most of you are simply looking for a safe space to be yourself.

This is why shifting the face of beauty means moving away from limited definitions and helping women find true beauty inside and out. Beauty is exactly what you already possess, and by finding it, you dare to redefine it and be at peace in your own skin—not just comfortably, but extravagantly, deeply, loudly, at the top of your lungs! This is true beauty. This is strength. This is power. And if you have that, it doesn't matter what's trending.

The Influence of Self-image on Skin Health

You know that confidence is a wonderful ingredient for a fulfilling life, but did you know that self-appreciation plays a central role in shaping your emotional well-being and physical health—specifically, your skin? Yes, how you see yourself, speak to yourself, and treat yourself all have a deep connection to how your skin looks and feels. This connection between your emotions and skin is called the psycho-dermatological connection or the skin-mind connection. Your skin really *does* look different depending on how you feel.

And science backs this up. Being overly self-critical causes stress, which means your body releases cortisol, triggering inflammation that leads to skin issues and sensitivity. But the power of the skin-mind connection lies in this truth: Positive thoughts and emotions, like self-compassion, listening to yourself, and confidence, promote the release of endorphins, which neutralize the harmful effects of cortisol, reducing inflammation and improving the health of your skin barrier. In a nutshell? Confidence makes you *stronger*.

Understanding Self-image

Pause here for a moment and consider these questions:

> *How do I see myself?*
>
> *What words do I use when I talk or think about my face, my skin, my presence in the world?*
>
> *Am I kind or am I harsh?*

The way you answer these questions matters more than you think. Your self-image—the mental picture you hold of who you are—touches every aspect of your life. The way you see yourself influences your emotions, your choices, your relationships, and the way you move through the world.

The problem with self-image is that it often doesn't matter how you look; it matters how you *feel* about how you look. It's a script that plays in your head every time you see your reflection or a photo of yourself. You can be *looking* at yourself, but you don't really *see* yourself. What you see is what you've been taught to see—and this has power.

3. THE PSYCHOLOGY OF BEAUTY

People with a positive self-image generally have higher self-esteem, which is linked to better mental health. On the other hand, a negative self-image—seeing yourself through a lens of judgment or lack—can manifest in physical ways, often leading to sometimes devastating conditions like body dysmorphia, eating disorders, or chronic skin issues like acne, eczema, or psoriasis.

But here's what matters most about your self-image: It's not static. It's ever-changing based on your experiences, your mood, and the way you engage with yourself. This is good news because it means you can reshape the relationship you have with yourself, even if you've spent decades disliking who you are. You have the power to intentionally nurture a healthy self-image, enhancing your emotional well-being and giving yourself permission to feel good about who you are, inside and out. You can create space for healing and confidence, and, ultimately, good skin health.

The Impact of Self-image on Mental Health and Skincare Routines

Your self-image doesn't just affect your emotional well-being; it also influences how you approach self-care—in this case, skincare. Think about your skincare routine. When you stand in front of the mirror, what thoughts surface? Do you take the time to look at yourself, to make eye contact with your reflection? Do you approach your routine with intention and care, like someone worthy of attention? Or do you rush through the process, half-present? Do you wash your face more aggressively than usual when you feel angry, sad, or frustrated? How you treat your skin can tell you a lot about how you're treating yourself.

When practiced with mindfulness and self-compassion, a skincare routine isn't about products. It's about being present with yourself, an act that nurtures both your skin and your spirit. Presence can transform your everyday routine into an extraordinary act of self-respect.

Try it: Next time you start your skincare routine, take a moment to look at yourself in the mirror. Don't magnify or zoom in on what you don't like or self-criticize, but practice *seeing* yourself.

Part of the universal human experience is how you choose to express yourself. You want to show up in the world in ways that pay tribute to your stories, to the complexity of your experiences, and to the ways you make meaning of your life. You approach most areas of your life in this way, so why shouldn't the way you show up for your skin also reflect this desire for expression? When you perform your skincare routine, you're telling your mind and body that your individuality is power and deserves to be expressed!

So much of your time as a woman is spent putting other people's needs first. Consistently spending time doing something significant for yourself—no matter how small—is not just a routine, it's a reminder that the way you take care of the needs of others can only ever be as effective as the way you take care of your own needs. And not making yourself an afterthought will lead to tangible improvements in your skin.

Skincare is a consistent practice, a habit that can ground you in your day and offer a sense of control over your environment. In times of stress or uncertainty, having a routine provides structure, reassurance, and comfort. And, over time, as you begin to see improvements in your skin health, you'll experience a deeper sense of accomplishment as a result of choosing yourself day after day.

The Emotional Impact of Achieving Skincare Goals

Achieving your skincare goals is deeply empowering. For many women entering their thirties and beyond, one of the most common concerns is premature aging. Most likely throughout your life, you were told to wear sunscreen daily, cover your face when outdoors, and use good-quality products. But few women have access to such products in their teens and twenties. Often it's only in your thirties that you may finally be in a position to buy these products after spending more than a decade wanting to do better for yourself, your health, and your skin.

By the time you're able to provide for yourself in the ways you've always wanted to—and deserved to—a lot of skin damage, like sun damage and stress, has likely already been done. So *finally* being able to take care of your skin can feel like it's already too late. But it's not. Being able to nourish and heal your skin is a representation of your story, of everything you have overcome to be where you are, and of the power you have to design the life *you want now*. You might be feeling hopeless at the signs of sun damage and premature aging, but there *is* a solution, and access to this information is no longer only for the privileged.

There are scientifically supported ingredients that *can* improve the signs of premature aging, and I've built my company and legacy on this truth. It's not too late to have the youthful complexion you worry you neglected for too long. Late nights of studying to achieve your dreams, juggling two jobs to pay your bills, sleepless nights while you raised your babies, and afternoons on the beach with your friends shouldn't be regrets. You shouldn't have to compromise making a living for life.

And my ultimate secret weapon for *reversing* the signs of aging is the heartbeat of Gin Amber Beauty: microneedling. I'll get more into this in Chapter 8, but for now, as part of your journey to better skin health and confidence, I want you to know that achieving your skincare goals is possible no matter what your story is. Being a woman in the world means experiencing high levels of stress *just to get by*. But you struggled, you overcame, and you made it here. Gin Amber Beauty is built for every woman, for every stage of life because what it's cost you to get where you are now shouldn't determine how you feel about who you are as a person. You've worked so hard to get here—you deserve skin that gives back to you.

Building a Healthy Relationship with Your Skin

Practicing your skincare routines and achieving your skincare goals is a message to your nervous system that you're *safe*. All relationships need safety and trust to bloom. Many women have faced challenges in life that have left them feeling like they aren't safe in their bodies, but building a healthy relationship with your skin is about taking that power *back*. Repetitive actions rewire your brain which, in turn, changes the way your nervous system communicates. Choosing you every single day heals the survival messages that have kept you in cycles of self-neglect and self-hatred, allowing you to open yourself up to everything life has to offer. Because beautiful skin is your birthright.

CHAPTER 4

BUILDING A SKINCARE ROUTINE

Now that you've explored the deeper layers of skincare, you can begin to move from the *why* to the *how*. In my experience, many questions about handling aging skin are universal.

How many skincare products do I need in my everyday routine?

What ingredients should I specifically be looking for based on my individual skincare concerns?

How often should I be doing a particular practice or using a product?

How can I target premature aging, dark spots, rosacea, acne, pigmentation?

What steps can I take to feel at home in my skin?

At heart, your skincare routine is a conversation with your skin. So building it must answer *your* questions while keeping the process realistic, accessible, and able to fit into your schedule. A healthy relationship with your skin and redefining body safety through daily acts of self-love and self-nurturance means intentionally setting aside time to care for yourself. But as a highly motivated, busy entrepreneur and mother myself, I understand better than anyone that a successful skincare routine must also include a realistic adaptation to your life and its responsibilities. Success in any area of life starts with making sure that you can consistently show up to take the necessary steps to achieve your goals. Your skin is no different. That's why the tools I've created through Gin Amber Beauty are intentionally simple and made to meet women where they are, not add more stress.

You might be worried that it's too late to start a skincare routine. I've worked with many women in their late thirties, forties, fifties, and beyond who are only now starting to prioritize better skin health. Perhaps you were told that taking care of yourself was selfish, or you didn't feel safe enough in your body to show up for yourself in a meaningful way until much later in life. I was one of these women. Or maybe you've been paralyzed because you just don't know where to start. Whatever your reason, know this: Starting today *counts*. Let me assure you that prioritizing your skin health can be simple—and it's never too late. So breathe. This chapter is your guide on where to start.

In keeping things uncomplicated, let's begin with the golden rule of skincare routine: You only need a handful of products every single day to bring out the natural best of your skin. And when I say handful, I mean handful! My golden rule is that you only need five essential products for a comprehensive, all-round daily skincare routine. So, what are they?

4. BUILDING A SKINCARE ROUTINE

Five Products Every Woman Needs for Healthy, Glowing Skin

Let's start with the basics. Every good skincare routine involves five essential products: makeup remover (when needed), a gentle cleanser, a serum, a moisturizer, and sunscreen. Now, let's unpack your ideal vanity case.

Makeup Remover

I'm mentioning makeup remover first because it's important to include it right at the start of your routine if you wear makeup. This step may not be for everyone, so if you don't wear makeup—every day or occasionally—you can jump to the next step.

Because not all cleansers are able to fully remove makeup, especially long-wear foundations and waterproof mascaras, skipping this step can leave residue behind that clogs pores and dulls your skin. So, gently remove makeup with a balm or oil before washing your face. This two-step cleanse will prevent a buildup of impurities and ensure your skin is always thoroughly cleansed.

Gentle Cleanser

A gentle cleanser is a non-negotiable foundation for skin health. It removes sweat, excess oil, pollution, and dead skin cells without damaging your skin barrier. Select a cleanser that is suitable for your skin type. You may pick a milky or gel cleanser, whatever you prefer. What's important are the ingredients and their suitability for your skin concerns.

Remember, I recommend only cleansing your face at night to protect your skin's natural balance. In the morning, you can start with your serums (the next step). Even if the instructions on your cleanser say to cleanse in the morning and at night, it's okay to skip the morning face wash. You will still reap the benefits; in fact, you'll likely experience more!

GIN AMBER BEAUTY PRO-TIP: Have a towel that you use exclusively for your face. Using a separate towel is important because it helps prevent the transfer of bacteria, oil, and dead skin cells from other parts of your body that can clog pores and trigger breakouts or irritation. The face is more delicate and sensitive, so reusing a body towel, especially one that's damp or used multiple times, can introduce unwanted microbes or harsh friction that compromises your skin barrier. A clean, dedicated face towel helps maintain better hygiene and supports healthier, clearer skin.

Serums

Serums are a must-have, especially for women over thirty. They're concentrated formulas packed with active ingredients that target specific skin concerns and penetrate deeper than moisturizers because of their smaller molecules, which is what makes them so powerful. They are also incredibly lightweight, making them ideal for everyday use. Don't be fooled by the size of their bottles—these little babies are liquid gold!

Once you've removed your makeup and cleansed your face, pat it dry with a clean towel and gently apply your serum. Follow the instructions of your specific product, but usually one or two drops is more than enough. If you're layering serums and other products, apply them based on consistency: from the most watery to the thickest. This ensures maximum product absorption.

Serum is best applied by patting it onto the skin with your fingertips rather than rubbing it in. This prevents you from pulling on your skin and compromising its elasticity. Remember, serums are highly concentrated; a little goes a long way—for your skin and for your wallet!

Moisturizer

Once you've applied your serum, it's time for your moisturizer. Moisturizers do exactly what the word suggests—they seal in moisture! Their job is to keep your skin hydrated and protected from drying out. Moisturizers also ensure all the goodness from your serum remains locked in. This is crucial for anti-aging.

4. BUILDING A SKINCARE ROUTINE

Sunscreen

Finally, don't forget to apply sunscreen to your morning routine. A non-nano mineral sunscreen with SPF 15 to 25 is sufficient for face protection, and ensures your body remains free of the nasties found in stronger SPFs and chemical sunscreens. UV rays are the number-one cause of premature aging, sun spots, hyperpigmentation, and skin cancer. Mineral sunscreens sit on the skin rather than being absorbed, so they offer more than enough protection for your skin needs. Any day that you spend significant time outdoors, remember to reapply every two hours or after sweating or getting out of water. Sunscreen not only protects against sun damage and skin cancer, it also protects against premature aging. This step alone can dramatically influence your skin health over the next ten years, especially if your sunscreen has active ingredients like peptides, like Gin Amber Beauty mineral sunscreen does.

Okay, now you have my simple five-step routine for more youthful, healthy skin. I want to add a sixth step, microneedling, which can be done as little as twice a week, perfect for those with busy schedules. But I'll go into this in more detail later. Microneedling involves its own steps, and I believe so much in this practice that I'm dedicating an entire chapter to it. So keep reading—it gets even better!

Actives: Peptides, Acids, and Vitamins

For now, let's learn about the building blocks of skincare.

Peptides

Peptides are amino acid chains (fragments of proteins) that communicate with your skin to produce more collagen. They are key for firming support. They're ideal for women experiencing a loss of elasticity or firmness, like those with aging skin. They're also great for overall skin repair.

Hyaluronic Acid

Hyaluronic acid is a must-have for hydration because it draws water into your skin. It can hold one thousand times its weight in water, making your skin plumper and smoother. Apply it to damp skin to achieve the best results, and then lock in the hydration with your moisturizer. This acid is ideal for women with dry, tight skin.

Niacinamide

Niacinamide is a buster for uneven skin tone and enlarged pores. Also known as vitamin B3, niacinamide soothes inflammation and reduces redness, assisting with dull, lifeless skin. It's ideal for anyone with sensitive or rosacea-prone skin as well as dark marks and uneven skin tone.

Vitamin C

Vitamin C is the most asked-about active ingredient in the skincare business. The reason? This is your skin's natural illuminator. And who doesn't want brighter, more radiant skin? The problem with vitamin C in many serums is that in order to achieve the ideal balance, the concentration of vitamin C needs to be perfect. Too low and it will be ineffective; too high and it will cause your skin to become irritated and sensitive, as well as vulnerable to sun damage.

As someone with sensitive skin, before creating Gin Amber Beauty, I spent years doing research on active ingredients. I've come to understand that there are different forms of vitamin C, and that if not used correctly, it will cause more harm than good.

When choosing a serum for skin brightening, be sure to read the ingredients carefully and choose the right concentration and form of vitamin C. The most common forms you'll find in serums are L-ascorbic acid, sodium ascorbyl phosphate, tetrahexyldecyl ascorbate, magnesium ascorbyl phosphate, or ascorbyl tetraisopalmitate. L-ascorbic acid is pure vitamin C and is very harsh in high concentrations (15–20 percent or greater). It should be avoided if you have sensitive skin or are using vitamin C for the first time.

Sodium ascorbyl phosphate, tetrahexyldecyl ascorbate, magnesium ascorbyl phosphate, and ascorbyl tetraisopalmitate are gentler and often better tolerated. They'll provide similar benefits without the potential for irritation. Avoid combining vitamin C with strong acids (AHAs/BHAs), benzoyl peroxide, or retinoids in the same routine to prevent irritation or reduced effectiveness.

Whichever serum you choose, remember to start slow and give your skin a chance to adjust. Some serums may even recommend that you only use vitamin C every other day and that you start gradually with the lowest concentration (below 10 percent), increasing frequency as your skin's tolerance improves. If you notice irritation, use the serum less regularly or stop altogether. It may be worth trying a different brand at this stage.

Vitamin C is also ideal for women with dark spots or pigmentation, which is one of the most common concerns in skincare. But not all pigmentation is the same, and different causes may require different approaches. For instance, sunspots or acne scars can often be addressed with vitamin C because it is known to lighten dark spots and protect against future damage. However, when it comes to hormonal pigmentation, such as melasma (often caused by pregnancy or hormonal changes), the solution is a bit more complex. Melasma isn't just an external issue; it's also due to internal hormonal imbalances. While topical treatments like vitamin C may help, the results won't be as effective as they would be for other forms of pigmentation.

Melasma may require more intensive treatments, including prescriptions like hydroquinone. But it's important to note that this isn't my first choice. Lifestyle changes to address the hormonal imbalance should be your first course of action. Hormonal pigmentation is tough to treat because it's often caused by increased cortisol levels or stress. Women release a significant amount of cortisol during childbirth, which could explain the melasma postpartum that many women experience. Because melasma also can be related to stress, managing stress and improving lifestyle choices, such as adopting a healthier diet and taking care of your skin holistically, are most definitely part of the answer.

The Complex World of Retinoids and Skincare Acids

The deeper I've gone into researching skincare, the clearer it's become. When it comes to retinoids and skincare acids, there is far more to consider than most people realize. Before I dive into this section, I want to offer a gentle note. My intention is not to scare you away from retinoids—they're one of the most well-researched and effective ingredients in skincare. The Gin Amber Beauty 2.5% retinol serum is part of my own skincare routine. That said, it's important to understand how to use retinoids effectively and safely because they're potent. This section is here to empower you with facts so you can make informed choices, avoid common pitfalls, and get the best results.

Tretinoin - There are many forms of retinoids like retinol, retinaldehyde, adapalene, and isotretinoin, but tretinoin (or retinoic acid/Retin-A) is the most potent form. Tretinoin is a prescription-strength form of vitamin A. In the retinoid family, it's one of the strongest topical forms. The reason it's so powerful is because it sheds dead skin cells and speeds up the growth of fresh, new skin. In short, it works.

But it has its downsides. Its potency means that it increases the likelihood of dryness, irritation, and sensitivity and thins skin's protective barrier.[7] Additionally, tretinoin is not suitable for pregnant or breastfeeding women. In fact, it is illegal for doctors to prescribe tretinoin to pregnant women. It can cross the placenta barrier and potentially lead to serious birth defects and lifelong complications.

This brings up a broader question: If tretinoin is so harmful to a fetus, what does it do to the rest of the body? Even for those who aren't pregnant, could it have long-term effects on the brain and other organs? It's a valid concern, especially given how easily tretinoin is absorbed into the skin and bloodstream. These are the kinds of questions researchers are still exploring, but they're worth keeping in mind when deciding whether to include tretinoin in your skincare routine.

Accutane - A well-known variation of tretinoin is isotretinoin, a chemotherapy agent created in the 1970s for people with skin cancer. Isotretinoin is the active ingredient in Accutane, an oral medication prescribed for severe cases

---

7. Lee, M. W. (2020). "The Detrimental Side Effects of Retinol: Beyond Beauty Products." *University Honors Theses*. Paper 895. doi.org/10.15760/honors.916

of acne, particularly cystic acne, which can be challenging to treat. It's highly effective but also highly controversial due to its side effects.

Accutane is so potent that if a woman becomes pregnant while taking it, doctors are required by law to advise termination because the risk of congenital disabilities is nearly 100 percent. In some countries, including the U.S., strict regulations around the use of Accutane include an obligatory pregnancy test and, at times, a requirement that women use two forms of birth control while taking it.

For teenagers and young adults who struggle with severe acne, Accutane can feel like a miracle drug. But it's not without its complications and side effects. Many people struggle with dry, cracked lips, thinning skin, and even long-term issues like liver damage. And while some dermatologists argue that the benefits outweigh the risks for those with severe acne, I suggest that you consider alternative treatments and holistic approaches that address the root causes of acne rather than relying solely on prescription drugs.

"Check your fridge" is what I often tell my clients. What you eat has so much to do with your gut bacteria, and I can tell a lot about a person's skin issues by simply looking at the contents of their fridge. The usual culprits are sugar, gluten, dairy, and processed foods. Try temporarily removing these from your diet and seeing if there's any improvement in your skin.

One of the more concerning aspects of Accutane, as well as other retinoic acids, is its potential impact on mental health. There have been numerous reports of people experiencing depression, anxiety, and even suicidal thoughts while taking Accutane.

For young people already struggling with the emotional stress of severe acne, adding a medication with potential mental health side effects can be dangerous. On one hand, clearing up skin can boost confidence and improve overall well-being. I can see how reverse-engineering the healing process by starting with something like Accutane and then following that up with my recommendations for product and lifestyle changes may be necessary for some women. On the other hand, the possibility of experiencing mental health issues while on the drug is a serious risk that shouldn't be overlooked. I understand the challenges of being a woman with debilitating insecurity because of your skin, but finding the right solution for your individual needs must be handled with full transparency, honesty, and the right support. You deserve to make empowered, informed choices about what goes onto your skin and into your body.

Retinol - Retinol is a derivative of vitamin A. It's widely regarded as the gold standard anti-aging agent, which is why it's most often found in serums for mature skin. It also helps with fine lines, dullness, and even breakouts. Retinol is a lot milder than retinoic acid but still delivers noticeable anti-aging effects. I recommend plant-based retinols, which are plant-derived alternatives to traditional vitamin A. These include bakuchiol, rosehip seed oil, and carrot seed extract.

Please note: Even though retinol is milder and more tolerable than retinoic acid, the risks during pregnancy are still there. Remember, my goal is not to alarm you with this information—retinol is safe when used correctly.

Our Gin Amber Beauty 2.5% retinol serum has been formulated to be effective yet gentle. We've combined plant-based retinol with soothing oils and antioxidants, and it is free from any irritants. I recommend using Gin Amber Beauty hyaluronic acid serum before the retinol serum to lock in moisture and soften the skin. Apply it at night followed by a non-nano mineral sunscreen the next day.

Salicylic Acid - Salicylic acid is another common ingredient in acne treatments for those with oily skin. It penetrates the pores and breaks down the excess sebum (oil) that can lead to blackheads, whiteheads, and pimples. Salicylic acid is often found in cleansers and spot treatments, which makes it an option for mild acne.

It's best to start with a low concentration and slowly increase as needed, paying attention to how your skin responds.

4. BUILDING A SKINCARE ROUTINE

The Dangers of Over-Exfoliation

One of the biggest mistakes people make with their skincare routines is over-exfoliating. Exfoliants include scrubs with sugar, salt, or microbeads, and tools like exfoliating sponges, gloves, or dermaplaning blades. They often think that the more they do, the better the results will be. But while exfoliating acids can help improve skin texture, using exfoliants too often can damage the skin's protective barrier. As mentioned before, this barrier helps to keep moisture in and harmful bacteria out, so when it is compromised, the skin becomes more susceptible to irritation, dryness, and infection.

Over-exfoliation can also lead to increased sensitivity and redness, and in some cases that I've seen, it can even cause breakouts when the skin tries to compensate for the loss of natural oils by producing more sebum. My advice is to avoid over-exfoliating altogether and to only use exfoliating acids and tools in moderation. For most people, exfoliating once a week is sufficient.

CHAPTER 5
CHRONIC SKIN ISSUES

Skin Issues and Holistic Treatments

It's important that I dedicate an entire chapter of this book to chronic skin issues. These conditions are frustrating, embarrassing, possibly painful, and, in my experience, they are deeply misunderstood. Like I've discussed, I believe holistic skincare approaches are the most effective form of treatment for any chronic skin condition. As such, understanding the conditions means going beyond topical application and exploring under the surface. Remember, your skin is telling a story of what's going on inside your body. Your job is to listen.

Rosacea

Many people treat rosacea like a rash—put some cream on it and wait for it to heal. But here's the truth: Rosacea is an autoimmune disorder that affects the skin, causing visible blood vessels, redness, a burning sensation, and even pain. It can be an extremely uncomfortable condition to live with because it's so painful and noticeable. Having struggled with rosacea for most of my life, I know the challenges of living with such an awkward condition. I remember crying when I looked in the mirror, frustrated that nothing I was trying at the time was working. I started to withdraw from social situations because I felt self-conscious and embarrassed.

There are different subtypes of rosacea, and depending on which type you suffer from, the treatments may differ slightly. Erythematotelangiectatic rosacea (ETR) is a mild form that causes persistent facial redness and flushing, including skin sensitivity and a stinging sensation. Heat, spicy foods, sun exposure, and alcohol are all triggers.

Papulopustular rosacea causes bumps and acne-like lesions. This subtype can co-occur with ETR and is extremely painful. It differs from acne because the lesions don't have blackheads or whiteheads, but they are sensitive and inflamed. Metronidazole is a prescription antibiotic that is typically applied topically to treat this subtype, but it can also be taken orally.

Phymatous rosacea, more common in men, causes thickened skin, especially on the nose. It also leads to enlarged pores and changes in skin texture.

When I first learned that the majority of people with rosacea have an overgrowth of H. pylori bacteria in their gut,[8] it was like a lightbulb went off. Up until that point in my life, I had been told there was no cure. But finding out that, in fact, there *was* something I could do about rosacea through the skin-gut connection was empowering. It explained why external treatments alone had never been enough and why it was so important for me to reassess my lifestyle at the time.

One of the biggest turning points in my skin healing journey was when I decided to cut out alcohol and coffee and follow a keto diet. Just these simple steps dramatically reduced my rosacea flare-ups, and, together with dermarolling, I can now confidently say that I've cured my rosacea. I no longer have painful flare-ups or embarrassing situations I can't control. If you're dealing with rosacea, I recommend cutting out dairy, gluten, refined sugar, processed foods, alcohol, and caffeine for ninety days. The results may surprise you.

---

8. Gao, Y., Yang, X. J., Zhu, Y., Yang, M., & Gu, F. (2024). "Association between rosacea and helicobacter pylori infection: A meta-analysis." *PLoS One*, 19(4), e0301703. doi: 10.1371/journal.pone.0301703

Be gentle with your skin when managing rosacea. Focus on soothing the skin, avoiding harsh exfoliants, and opting for products that are mild and nourishing. Incorporate vitamin C into your regimen to benefit from its anti-inflammatory properties, which can help calm the redness and inflammation associated with rosacea. If you're ready to go one step further, microneedling is another tool that has proven to be safe and effective for managing rosacea. But remember, *all* skincare routines and healing processes take time, so consistency and patience are pivotal during the healing practices.

These simple approaches combined with inward lifestyle changes, such as diet, gut health, therapy to address emotional struggles or suppressed feelings, and stress management are key to improving your symptoms. Many women underestimate the effect emotional stress can have on their skin health. *Any* stress can increase cortisol and inflammation in your body, so getting to the root of why you feel stressed is important. The human body is a work of art; if you can learn to appreciate the connection you have with how it functions, you'll find the power to change your life and your skin health.

Eczema and Psoriasis

Just like with rosacea, eczema and psoriasis are more than just dry, flaky skin. It can be very tempting to rely solely on ointments and creams, especially because it requires very little effort to use them. But sometimes you have to take a deeper look at what is causing the issue to stop it. Eczema and psoriasis are often rooted in issues with gut health or parasites. I found that simple detox worked wonders for my skin. Simply removing coffee, dairy, and sugar from my diet radically transformed not only my skin's appearance, but my relationship with my skin and my body overall. And detoxifying your body does *not* have to be complicated. Fermented foods like kimchi, sauerkraut, and naturally fermented pickles are fantastic for your gut and incredibly simple to incorporate into your life. You can even make your own!

If fermented foods aren't your thing, a high-quality probiotic supplement is a great alternative. The more you focus on internal healing, the less you'll have to rely on external solutions.

Melasma

Melasma is a common skin condition that causes dark, discoloured patches on the skin, especially the face. It usually appears on the cheeks, forehead, upper lip, and bridge of the nose. Melasma occurs when the pigment-producing cells in your body, also called the melanocytes, become overactive and produce too much melanin, the pigment that gives skin its color. There are a few common triggers for melasma, including sun exposure, hormonal changes like pregnancy or the use of birth control, and even heat and inflammation.

Effectively managing melasma requires a consistent combination of approaches that include sun protection as the foundation. I always say, the first step is to protect! Melasma is harmless, but it can be persistent and difficult to treat. Consistent use of toxic-free sunscreen combined with antioxidants and brightening or repair creams formulated specifically for pigmentation concerns, like Gin Amber Beauty 10% vitamin C + squalene repair cream, are your best allies. Microneedling is also an incredibly effective way to help control melasma, but your first line of defense is daily, toxic-free mineral sunscreen!

Acne

Acne is most often traced back to hormonal changes, especially during puberty. Changes in androgen, or steroid hormone, levels in the body stimulate excess sebum (oil) production. This excess oil can clog pores and lead to breakouts. But from a holistic standpoint, just like anything that's happening on your skin, acne is also a reflection of what's going on inside your body. A diet high in processed foods, sugar, gluten, and dairy can contribute to inflammation and acne. Poor gut health and bad sleep habits have also been linked to acne—so no wonder this most often plagues teenagers!

5. CHRONIC SKIN ISSUES

A holistic approach that addresses both the internal and topical factors that cause acne is best when it comes to managing and treating it. Balancing your hormones through stress management and good gut health along with using topical treatments like Gin Amber Beauty natural AHA/BHA exfoliating cleanser and vitamin C serum to gently cleanse your skin without stripping its natural, healthy oils will create harmony inside your body, leading to clearer, healthier skin.

Gut Health

When thinking about holistic skin health, it helps to remember that your skin often mirrors the condition of your gut. One approach that many find supportive is the GAPS protocol, created by Dr. Natasha Campbell-McBride. Rather than focusing only on surface-level treatments, GAPS begins by nourishing the digestive system, working in three stages: an introductory phase with soothing foods such as bone broths and fermented juices; a full diet rich in nutrient-dense staples like meats, eggs, healthy fats, and probiotic foods; and finally a gradual reintroduction of other whole foods once balance is restored. The intention is to reduce irritants, repair the gut lining, and rebalance the microbiome so the body can naturally detoxify and heal—changes that are often mirrored in the skin's clarity and resilience. The GAPS philosophy highlights an important truth for anyone seeking radiant skin: When you nurture the gut, the skin often follows.

Detox and Colonics

Let's talk detox. I know it's become a bit of a buzzword in today's culture, but there really are benefits to understanding this concept. Toxins build up in the body simply from everyday living in a modern world, and these toxins can eventually cause disruptions. Regular removal of this toxic buildup allows your body to do what it does naturally, like healing, without any interference.

When I was deep in my own skincare journey, I committed to weekly colonics for a year. Colonics, or colon hydrotherapy, are a cleansing procedure designed to flush the large intestine (colon) with warm, filtered water to remove built-up waste, mucus, and toxins. It wasn't glamorous, but it was effective, not just for my skin but for my overall health. Regular colonics improve digestion, enhance nutrient absorption, offer relief from constipation, increase energy, and improve skin health. I saw dramatic progress in my digestion and skin health. Remember, addressing chronic skin issues is all about healing from the inside out.

Colonics are generally considered safe when performed by a qualified practitioner. A colonic is similar to an enema, except that colonics involve much larger volumes of water to flush the entire colon, not just the lower part of the colon, which is the purpose of an enema.

When to See a Dermatologist

No matter what the issue—pigmentation, rosacea, eczema, or psoriasis—topical treatments usually only ever address the symptoms, not the cause. Traditional dermatologists can prescribe medicated creams that can temporarily soothe irritation, but unless you explore what else is going on with your body and your mental health, the issue will more than likely keep coming back. As I said before, skin issues are often a reflection of what's happening internally, so focusing on the cause is the closest you'll ever get to a cure—not just a band-aid for symptoms.

That being said, there is absolutely a time and place for dermatologists, especially when it comes to skin cancer, questionable-looking moles, or inflammation that is painful or uncontrolled. If you're a sun lover or if you've noticed something concerning on your skin, a visit to your dermatologist can be lifesaving. My work and this book are not about relying only on natural and alternative remedies at the risk of overlooking potentially harmful skin situations; rather, I am advocating for having *all* of the options available to you. Melanoma is one of the easiest cancers to treat if caught in time, so regular mole checkups will give you not just peace of mind, but validation that you're successfully caring for your own body. True prevention and overall well-being is all about consistent, healthier habits, including self-sufficiency.

It's okay to acknowledge that taking care of yourself can sometimes seem scary. Perhaps it's not a behavior that was modelled by your own mother or caregiver. Moreover, most women are encouraged to consider themselves *last*. Be the good girl, right? But true feminine power lies in understanding that you're allowed to take care of yourself. You don't need to be scared—whatever you have to face, you will face with your head held high knowing that you can trust *you*. You're healing the relationship you have with your skin and your soul; you're turning the lens of compassion and reflection back toward your own heart and listening to your inner voice. If you've put off seeing a dermatologist, or any doctor for that matter, because you're scared of what you might find out, this is your reminder that you deserve to be taken care of. This is your reminder that you're safe. This is your reminder of the supernatural power of the body to bend, break, and heal. You're so much more than you've given yourself credit for up until now, and you will survive whatever this day brings.

Simple Changes, Real Results

What I love about the work I do with women and the message I try to share with the world through my products and content is this: Real solutions are simple. You don't need twelve different products twice a day, infinite time, or the latest trend. You just need a clean, consistent routine with toxic-free ingredients and the courage to cut out things that are harming you. Simple changes, like cutting out coffee, alcohol, refined sugar, and processed food, can be difficult at first. I know because I've been there! I had headaches and withdrawal symptoms when I first made these changes to my life, but no matter how difficult it was to persevere on the hard days, I was no longer willing to accept mediocre health for my skin or my body. I'd followed the world's trends all my life, and none of them had brought me closer to the version of myself I wanted to be. But like with all hard things, the headaches passed, the hard days came less often, and I started to connect with the voice that had quietly been residing within all along. And now, my skin thanks me for making these choices. I didn't die without them; in fact, I feel better, younger, and healthier than I ever have in my life—and I'm forty!

Gin Amber Beauty and the work that I do is not about quick fixes or miracle cures. It's about something real. Through my brand, my products, and the way I live my life, my message to you is simple: *You have the power to change your life*. You don't need to be rich or well-connected; you don't need to have access to the most exclusive salons or wellness clinics; you don't need to wait until a better time or be younger or older or a better version of yourself. The power is already within you. All it asks from you is the courage to start.

CHAPTER 6

PROMOTING HEALTHY SKIN FROM THE INSIDE

In case I haven't said it enough, let me say it again: Healthy skin starts from within! There's an energetic connection between your skin and your nervous system, your unresolved trauma, and your emotions. Your skin is an extension of these. Let's unpack this a bit.

Trauma and Emotional Healing

Unresolved trauma—whether from childhood, adulthood, or passed down through generations—can and often does manifest in physical ways, including on your skin. Dr. Gabor Maté, in his groundbreaking book *When the Body Says No*,[9] explores how stress, repressed emotions, and unresolved trauma impact the body. He makes a compelling case for how the body says "no" when you override your emotional needs, suppress emotions, and push yourself too far. This directly aligns with what I've observed in my work and experienced in my personal life. Just like other organs, when you ignore your emotional wounds or live in a chronic state of stress, your skin will

---

9. Maté, G. (2003). *When the Body Says No: The Cost of Hidden Stress*. Vintage Canada.

reflect the pain you're carrying. Maté says that chronic stress and emotional suppression lead to a dysregulation of your nervous and hormonal systems; often you are not even consciously aware of this. I've seen it, felt it, and lived it.

During a breathwork session I once attended, I experienced something I will never forget. As I lay there breathing deeply, I suddenly felt a wave of emotion flow through me and out of my body. I released something very tangible I didn't even know I was holding in that moment, and nothing I have ever done before or since as part of my healing has given me the same sense of release. I felt liberated from something ethereal, something I couldn't name or tame. All around me, people were crying, shaking, releasing lifetimes of trauma and tension. This is the power of somatic practices; they bypass the intellectual mind and access emotions stored in the physical body, bringing psychic awareness to them and giving them space to emerge, which allows you to let go.

I've seen powerful healing through breathwork practices. While you must be careful with claims, it's important for me to mention that some people have had life-altering experiences through this kind of work. Maté's book is evidence of this. The mind-body connection is real, and your skin is part of this communication.

Somatic Practices and the Nervous System

Your nervous system is at the center of your mind-body connection. Stress dysregulates this system, and chronic stress causes your body to remain in this dysregulated state constantly—this is known as the fight-or-flight state. In this state, your body prioritizes survival over healing. It will do whatever it must to survive your current environment and sacrifice any rest or repair it needs. Your body, including your skin, develops illness and inflammation as a result. Regulating your nervous system through practices like breathwork acts as a reset. Every time you do these practices, you shift your body from the fight-or-flight state into the rest-and-repair state of the parasympathetic nervous system. This is how you open the door for healing your skin. Your body is meant to heal itself, and somatic practices help activate that primal response. If you've never tried any, they're simple,

6. PROMOTING HEALTHY SKIN FROM THE INSIDE

free, and incredibly effective ways to support your mental, emotional, and skin health.

Breathwork, meditation, intentional visualization, and manifestation are all somatic practices that are free, accessible, and incredibly effective for calming your nervous system and, therefore, your skin.

Breathwork, Meditation, Visualization, and Manifestation for Healing

If meditation feels intimidating, know that you don't need to be able to sit still in one position for hours in order to experience its benefits. Start small. Even just ten to fifteen minutes a day can make a huge difference on your mind-body connection. In the morning, try breathwork to activate your body and mind for the day. My favorites are the breathing exercises developed by Wim Hof, also known as "The Iceman." Through controlled hyperventilation and breath retention, he created a three-step practice that reduces inflammation, manages stress, and promotes healing. You can search "Wim Hof breathing" on YouTube for videos to try at home.

In the evening, meditate to wind down and center yourself. Personally, I'm a huge fan of Dr. Joe Dispenza, whose work is freely accessible online. His work on meditation and neuroscience is fascinating. He's proven that by calming the mind, balancing the nervous system, and visualizing healing, you can actually change your brain's wiring and even alter your genes.

When I was healing from rosacea, I followed Dispenza's techniques religiously. Every morning and night I meditated, visualizing my skin as clear, healthy, and glowing. I didn't just sit there passively—I *felt* what my skin would look and feel like. Over time, my skin responded to this mindfulness. It healed. I manifested it!

Manifesting is the result of visualization. When you visualize your skin being healthy or when you set an intention to heal, you're telling your brain and body what you want. You *believe* in the possibility of change. But here's the catch: You can't just sit around hoping. You have to take aligned action.

Here's what this looks like practically: When you visualize your skin being healthy, act like it's already happened. What would a person with healthy skin do? What would that version of *you do?* Would you eat more nourishing food, prioritize healthy sleep, manage stress, or set boundaries with people who drain your energy? Would you attend therapy to uncover and work through the emotional pain that's holding you back from healing? Yes! Every small step must move you toward your goal with intention and action.

If you're dealing with a chronic skin condition, start by visualizing it as healed. Research what foods and products can support your skin, and find a routine that works for you. Set boundaries, make time for self-development, start exercising. All these steps will help reinforce what you're manifesting. When you take a small step in one area of your life, you teach your mind that goals are achievable in *every* area of your life, and you set a healthy cycle of intention, action, and healing in motion.

Physical Healing From the Inside Out

Once you begin to address the emotional roots—whether through therapy, self-development, or somatic practices—you create space in your life for deeper healing. From here, you can explore and incorporate physical changes that support healing from the inside out.

The Importance of Fats

There is much misinformation in the world about diets generally and diets in relation to skin health in particular. And fats are usually at the top of the list when it comes to food that is considered *bad*. You've been taught for decades to fear fats—that you should opt for low-fat everything. But here's the thing: Fats are, in fact, *essential* for an optimized system, including good skin health.

You need fat to absorb key nutrients like vitamin D and other fat-soluble vitamins. Even if you spend all day in the sun, without enough fat in your diet, your body can't absorb the vitamin D it needs.

6. PROMOTING HEALTHY SKIN FROM THE INSIDE

The right fats—especially from pasture-raised animals—are incredibly nourishing. Cows that are free to graze in the sun and eat grass produce the healthiest fats, which, in turn, support your hormones, brain, and yes, even your skin.

How Climate and Environment Affect Your Skin

Did you know that your climate of origin can influence the way your body processes certain food? Depending on where you were born, the climate you were raised in affects the type of food and nutrients your body needs.

People from northern, colder climates thrive on diets rich in animal fats, while people from warmer, more tropical climates naturally need fewer animal fats and more plant-based (therefore water-based) foods. The logic is simple. Animal fats keep you warm; fruits and veggies cool you down! Based on these needs, when you optimize your diet, you optimize your skin health.

This is yet another example of the wisdom of your body. Try adjusting your diet according to your ancestry and see how your skin improves.

Hydration

Dry skin isn't just an external issue—it's a sign that something is missing in your body. This is one you've heard before: When it comes to skin health, water is key. But that's not the whole story. Just because you drink a lot of water doesn't mean you're always hydrated. True hydration includes minerals and electrolytes, and, without them, your body can't hold the water you're drinking. In fact, without them, you may actually be causing harm by flushing out key nutrients that are already in your body. This is the risk of overhydration, which can impact your skin because your body needs more than just water to be hydrated.

Include mineral-rich foods, like leafy greens, good-quality Himalayan salt, Celtic salt, and fish, in your diet. And pay attention to your water source—spring or mineral water with trace elements is ideal. Use a good water filtration system at home if you need to. When you're properly nourished, your skin will show it.

Vitamin D and Sunlight

Sunlight plays an indispensable role in skin health. You've probably been conditioned to think that the sun is harmful, but the truth is the sun—especially early morning and late afternoon sun—is incredibly beneficial for your skin. It provides your body with vitamin D, which helps keep your immune system and skin healthy. Sunlight also helps with cell rejuvenation and collagen production, essential for smooth skin. So if you're afraid of spending time in the sun, especially if you're a woman over forty, I understand! But consider getting fifteen to thirty minutes of sunlight when UV rays aren't high—generally before 10:00 am and after 4:00 pm. This strength of sunlight isn't dangerous and is a vital part of healthy aging. And, as long as it's during those hours, you don't even need to wear sunscreen. I go on a morning stroll with my baby every day without any sunscreen on my face—and I soak up the beauty of warm sunshine on my skin! Morning sunlight exposure also helps improve your sleep-wake cycles, and the better your sleep, the better your skin repairs during the night.

Vitamin D is also available as a supplement. Just remember, vitamin D is a fat-soluble vitamin, meaning you need to consume it with fat for your body to absorb it properly. Eggs, especially the yolk, are a great source of fat that helps with vitamin D absorption. Without the right fat in your diet, you could be wasting your time and money on supplements. It's about getting the balance right.

Work-life Balance and Skin

Finally, don't underestimate the power of rest. Your work-life balance has a significant impact on your skin too. Skin repairs itself while you sleep, and if you're not getting quality rest, stressing too much, or burning out, no cream or serum will be able to compensate for that. Deep, restorative sleep is crucial for your skin's natural renewal process.

Circadian rhythm is your body's natural, internal twenty-four-hour clock that regulates sleep, hormones, digestion, and other essential bodily functions. Your body takes cues from light, particularly sunlight, on when to wake and when to rest. Early morning exposure to light signals your body to stop producing melatonin (the sleep hormone) and increase cortisol

6. PROMOTING HEALTHY SKIN FROM THE INSIDE

(which helps you wake up and feel alert). As the light fades in the evening, your body produces melatonin again to help you wind down and prepare for sleep.

Understanding your circadian rhythm and how you can support your body in its natural patterns is crucial for achieving deep, restorative sleep—and consequently improving the health of your skin.

Sleep is the most underrated beauty tool you have—and it's free. I know that parenting, relationships, work, self-care, and building your empire take their toll. As a woman of forty, I know that restful, restorative sleep has been a luxury up to now. But like with all things skin health, it's never too late to start. Waking up for babies at night and staying up late to study have all paid off; now is the time for you to prioritize rejuvenation. Be cautious about striving to be "strong" in the sense that "strong" means you're impervious to fatigue and feel guilty when you try to rest. "Strong" doesn't mean unbreakable. It means you listen to your own wisdom about when to work, when to push, when to stop, and when to rest. It means knowing how to put broken pieces back together in new ways. It means trusting that guidance comes not only from striving, but also from slowing down. You've earned it.

Supplements for Health and Anti-aging

I'm often asked: Do supplements actually work? Should I take them? What should I take? The short answer to all of these questions is yes—if you choose the right ones. Supplements are a great way to optimize your health without breaking the bank on high-end procedures. I regularly take nicotinamide mononucleotide (that's a mouthful, so let's just call it NMN), resveratrol, and nitric oxide. These are the cornerstones of my supplement routine.

My mom suffered from arthritis for years. She tried everything to manage the pain, but had accepted that this was just how things were going to be for her. Once I started using supplements, particularly the three I mentioned, I suggested that she also try them. After only six weeks, she called me in tears, exclaiming, "I don't have pain anymore!" She couldn't believe the difference, and honestly, neither could I. I mean I knew they were good, but not that good!

These supplements work by targeting aging and inflammation at a cellular level. NMN is particularly known for supporting DNA repair and has been extensively researched by Harvard professor David Sinclair, who spent twenty years researching NMN, resveratrol, and NAD+ specifically and aging and the body's ability to regenerate in general. He eventually authored the book *Lifespan*,[10] where he discusses his research. I base my recommendations as well as my personal supplement choices on this book. Sinclair advocates for the power of these supplements to slow the aging of cells, boost energy, and restore vitality.

While resveratrol comes naturally from grapes or red wine, for significant benefits, you'll want to supplement. It's all about giving your body the tools to renew itself.

Nitric oxide plays a critical yet often overlooked role in skin health and visible aging. As a powerful vasodilator, nitric oxide ensures that blood, oxygen, nutrients, and hydration reach every cell—including those deep within the skin. This molecule is produced by every cell in the body, but its production declines by about 10–12 percent each decade starting in your early twenties. By the time you reach your forties or fifties, you may be producing just half of what you once did. This drop significantly impacts the skin's ability to repair itself, generate collagen, and maintain its youthful elasticity and glow. Beyond natural aging, common medications such as NSAIDs, antibiotics, statins, proton pump inhibitors, and even antiseptic mouthwash can further suppress nitric oxide production, leaving most people in a state of deficiency without realizing it.

Dr. Nathan Bryan, a biochemist with over twenty years of research in nitric oxide science, developed a nitric oxide activating serum that brings groundbreaking innovation to skincare. This is the first age-defying skincare formula based on a Nobel Prize-winning discovery, designed not just to treat

---

10. Sinclair, D. A., & LaPlante, M. (2019). *Lifespan: Why We Age—and Why We Don't Have To*. Atria Books.

surface wrinkles but to correct their root cause: a lack of nitric oxide. When applied, the serum stimulates natural collagen production and restores the vital circulation of oxygen and nutrient-rich blood to skin cells, working at a deep cellular level to rejuvenate aging skin.

Advanced Therapies

The following advanced therapies were transformative in my own healing journey.

Ozone IV Therapy - Let's start with ozone therapy. Ozone IV therapy is one of the most revitalizing therapies I've ever experienced. It works by infusing your blood with ozone, a form of oxygen, which helps boost oxygen levels throughout your body. More oxygen in your body means stronger immunity, more energy, and clearer skin. When I first tried it, I felt an immediate boost in energy, and over time, I saw improvements in my skin as well. If you're considering it, start slow because too much ozone too quickly can overwhelm your body. But done correctly, the benefits are powerful.

Stem Cell Therapy - Stem cells are another powerful therapy gaining attention. Stem cells are cells in the body that have the potential to develop into many different types of cells, and as such, they're potent for healing. They rejuvenate and repair cells, helping heal skin and other organs. You can get stem cell treatments through IVs or even microneedling with stem cells for the face. It's an exciting and promising area of natural medicine. However, it's crucial to know where the stem cells come from. If you're getting a stem cell treatment, ask your provider where they source them. You want to be sure you're getting clean, ethically-sourced stem cells.

While these therapies are powerful, they can be costly. Ozone IVs aren't too expensive, but stem cell treatments can range from US$2,000 to US$3,000 and up to US$20k per session! But the results can be life-changing; so if you can afford them, they're worth considering.

Colonics and Enemas - I've discussed gut health quite a bit already, so by now I am sure you are aware of the importance of your inner ecosystem and its connection to your skin. A healthy gut simply means a healthier, clearer complexion.

One of the best ways to support your gut is through colonics. A colonic is a procedure where filtered, temperature-controlled water is slowly introduced into the colon through a tube inserted into the rectum.

Regularly cleansing the colon, specifically the large intestine, can help remove built-up waste and toxins, which improves not just your digestion but your skin as well. I used to suffer from terrible migraines, and nothing helped. But after I started doing regular colonics, the migraines completely disappeared. That's how impactful colonics were for me.

But don't overdo it. Start with once or twice a month and then increase to once a week. But listen to your body and how it responds and makes you feel. If you're adventurous, coffee enemas are also an option for gut cleansing. They go deeper than regular colonics, helping to detox the liver. But if you're just starting out, I recommend water-based colonics until your body is used to the process. It's not comfortable, but few things in healing are. If you want something different, you have to do something different.

So, if you're struggling with your skin, I encourage you to start with yourself—your thoughts, your emotions, and your body's needs. Get curious about what your body is telling you. Respond with love, patience, and empowerment. Healing takes time, but with the right tools and mindset, it's absolutely possible.

CHAPTER 7

SKINCARE THROUGH THE AGES

S kin is your lifelong companion. It changes as you do—shifting in resilience and needs depending on what phase of life you're in. So what does skin need at each stage of life?

Baby's First Skin

From birth, skin is an extraordinary organ. It begins forming four weeks into gestation and ensures that the fetus develops in a sterile environment. It forms in a way that protects the fetus from prolonged exposure to a watery home. Fascinating!

In the womb, a baby's skin is protected from amniotic fluid by a white substance covering it called vernix. It also allows a baby to move smoothly through the birth canal. After birth, vernix serves as a natural moisturizer and protective layer for a baby's delicate body while adjusting to life outside the womb for the first time. Hospitals often remove vernix right after a baby is born, but it's packed with good bacteria, and the longer it stays on a baby's skin after birth, the more beneficial its nutrients are for skin health over the person's lifetime. This is why I chose to birth my son at home—so that I could choose to leave vernix on.

A baby's skin is extremely sensitive; it's thinner and more absorbent than adult skin. It's still maturing, so it's more sensitive to irritants, allergens, and chemicals. Anything applied to a baby's skin is more easily absorbed into their bloodstream, making them more vulnerable to inflammation and imbalances in their bodies. This is why it's essential to choose products that are fragrance-free, gentle, and specially formulated for their delicate skin and whole-body health.

Another fascinating fact? More and more doctors recommend delaying cutting the umbilical cord for at least an hour after birth, allowing stem cells and vital nutrients more time to absorb into a baby's body. This provides a baby's immune system—and their skin—with a major head start in life. So if you're pregnant now or hoping to be pregnant in the future, or even if you know someone who could benefit from this knowledge, give the baby the opportunity for a lifetime of superior health. It really does start on day one.

Changing Skin

Okay, so it's likely that you were not lucky enough to benefit from extended time with your vernix or your umbilical cord. Now you have to protect and repair your skin from life in the world and often from a lifetime of bad skin choices. This isn't your fault. You inherited most of your knowledge from your parents or family, and you can only work with what you have.

This next section is for teenagers reading this book (or mothers with a teenager). You want to know: What can I do to help my skin now?

Teenage Skin: What's Really Going On?

For many, the teenage years are when first skin problems, like acne, start to appear. But acne isn't just a rite of passage or hormonal inevitability that you have to endure. It's often a reflection of deeper health or lifestyle issues.

Yes, teenagers go through hormonal changes, but the body is designed to handle those shifts. If your skin is generally healthy, occasional pimples are normal as your body adjusts to these changes. However, when acne becomes chronic and painful, it's a sign that something else—often related to diet, stress, and overall lifestyle—is out of balance. Even screen time can have an effect on skin. And during the teenage years, there's no shortage of any of these!

Remember: What you put into your body and what you're exposed to in your environment shows up on your skin. Stress and cortisol from adolescent social pressures, insecurity, hormonal changes due to puberty, and a general appeal for more independence (hello, fast food!) mean the teenage years are crammed with chaos. Combine that with living in front of screens and a potentially sedentary lifestyle, and it's a recipe for problematic skin.

Many people don't know that excessive screen time actually increases the skin's exposure to high-energy visible blue light, which penetrates the skin more deeply than the sun's UVB rays. This prolonged, close-up exposure leads to free radical damage, which breaks down collagen and increases inflammation. As of October 2025, on average, teenagers spend up to seven hours a day in front of their screens.[11] That's almost one-third of every day of their lives! That's more time than most adults spend in the sun over a week. It highlights just how much damage can be done and how powerful a simple change, like reducing screen time, can have on long-term skin health. That goes for everyone!

---

11. Duarte, F. (2025). "Average Screen Time for Teens (2025)." *Exploding Topics*. explodingtopics.com/blog/screen-time-for-teens

Skincare for Teens

Of course, a good skincare routine matters too. For teens, ingredients like salicylic acid can help unclog pores and soothe inflammation. It is also a superpower against occasional breakouts. But if your acne is severe and persistent, salicylic acid alone won't solve the problem; you need a more holistic approach.

In some cases, a dermatologist may prescribe treatments for chronic acne like Accutane, which can be very effective, especially in situations where your self-esteem and mental health are being impacted by your skin. It can be challenging to find the courage or motivation to make lifestyle changes when suffering from depression or anxiety fuelled by insecurity from chronic skin issues like acne. Starting with something like Accutane to feel better externally will allow you to heal the other internal factors impacting your mental health. In these cases, Accutane can be lifesaving. However, it should always be taken with caution, like I discussed in Chapter 5.

Accutane can have long-term side effects, particularly for girls. It can cause birth defects if you become pregnant, even after stopping the medication. It also disrupts menstruation and can cause hormonal imbalances. By now, you understand the severe impact these interferences can have on your skin. It is also known for excessively drying out lips, eyes, and skin, and dramatically increases skin sensitivity, which can continue long after the treatment ends. Accutane also has the potential for depression and aggravating existing mental health conditions, so if you (or someone you love) is considering Accutane, be sure to talk to your mental health care provider first. At the end of the day, it's only a temporary solution, and once you stop, if you haven't addressed the root cause of acne, it will come back even worse.

This is not designed to scare you or put you off medication like Accutane, but I'm a firm believer in the philosophy that knowledge is power, and you have the right to make informed choices about what goes into your body. Review all the information about Accutane—or any other medication for that matter—before you make your decision. You have the right to explore all of your options, including reaching out to me for help!

The Pill and Teenage Skin

In some cases, doctors prescribe birth control pills to teen girls for acne control, but this approach doesn't treat the root cause; it only masks the symptoms. I've seen it many times with girls I work with. At first, it seems like it's working—clearer skin, less oil. But once they stop taking the pill, many girls find that their breakouts return, often worse than before. This is because the pill doesn't address the causes of the hormonal imbalances or lifestyle factors that were the source of the breakouts in the first place. The key to healing teenage skin is not the medication—it's working from the inside out. It takes commitment, but it works. The earlier you tune into your skin and your healing, the stronger and healthier you'll be.

Skin and Pregnancy

When it comes to pregnancy, the skin can act similarly to how it does during the teenage years. Hormones are all over the place, and cravings can lead to poor food choices that affect your skin. During my pregnancy, I craved sugar and junk food and often gave into those cravings, and my skin broke out as a result. It wasn't just the pregnancy hormones; it was the bad diet. Once I got back to eating healthily, my skin improved.

As for skincare during pregnancy, you don't need to change much, but avoid prescription products and retinoids, including retinol. Everything else you were using before should be fine. Microneedling and vitamin C are safe and effective ways to manage pregnancy-related pigmentation issues too.

"Mature" Skin

I think it's safe to say that for women over thirty, something in your skin starts to change. Even though "midlife" is technically forty-five to sixty these days, most women experience visible shifts in their thirties, some even in their late twenties.

Goodbye Collagen

From the age of twenty-five, your collagen production starts to slow down. I know, I know—twenty-five! It sounds really young. And it is, but remember, hormones play a powerful role in skin health, and from the age of twenty-five, estrogen in your body starts to decline and so does the human growth hormone, both of which help your body to regenerate and heal.

You lose roughly one percent of collagen a year after the age of thirty. From an evolutionary perspective, at twenty-five, women are considered to be beyond reproduction and growth, and although the environment and society no longer reflect this, the ancient wisdom of the body is yet to adapt. When it comes to perimenopause and menopause, the shifts are even deeper. Hormonal changes are more dramatic during this time, with significant drops in estrogen and progesterone, which impact your skin health.

Botox and Fillers

So, from your thirties onward, your skin is considered "mature." This is when the aging starts. Fine lines and pigmentation are usually the first signs. This is the age when a lot of women begin thinking about Botox and fillers. In fact, many women these days start even earlier—as young as their early twenties. Now, I'm not here to judge what you do or do not do to take care of yourself and what makes you feel good about the way that you look. I did Botox and lip fillers to try to improve my appearance and my overall confidence, so I'm not telling you *not* to do Botox or fillers. But if these form part of your regular beauty practices, or you've considered starting, it's important to have all the information about these tools before utilizing them. It's also important to note that there *are* safer alternatives, and I'm going to get to that in the next chapter. (Yes, I'm talking about microneedling again!)

Here's the truth about Botox. It's glorified as the best way to stop aging, but Botox is a neurotoxin—yes, a toxin—that temporarily paralyzes your facial muscles. So, when you inject it into your forehead or around your eyes, for example, those areas stop moving, which means fewer wrinkles. But remember, this is *temporary*, and repeatedly paralyzing muscles with toxins can cause irreversible damage. The problem with Botox, and even with fillers, is that your facial muscles and skin get lazy. If you keep doing it over and over, you're teaching your face how not to function naturally. This means that when you rely on Botox, your skin stops doing the work.

7. SKINCARE THROUGH THE AGES

Additionally, if you aren't working with a properly-trained practitioner, they might inject you in the wrong place. You could end up with droopy brows and eyelids! Botox injections don't stimulate collagen production or change the nature of your skin. They simply mask the signs of aging.

Fillers, on the other hand, are less toxic, but they are still foreign substances injected directly into your skin. Most contain hyaluronic acid, which your body naturally produces, to plump the skin. While they sometimes produce impressive short-term results, clear long-term research is yet to confirm what the consequences will be down the line. Promoters of fillers claim that they eventually dissolve, but as of 2025, research suggests that hyaluronic acid fillers actually expand and retain water anywhere from two to fifteen years post-injection—*enlarging* the filler—which can migrate under the skin and result into a puffy face.[12]

Neither Botox nor fillers stimulate collagen production, unlike micro-needling, which is natural and proven to do so. So, while Botox and fillers may seem like a quick fix, they're training your skin to depend on them. Once you start, you have to keep doing them. Over time, this will change the structure of your face, and your skin will look *worse*. It sags, loses its youthful bounce, and is filled with toxins that can stay in your skin for *up to fifteen years*.

I've been there. I know what it feels like to be desperate for a quick fix, for something that will instantly improve the appearance of your skin and help you feel more confident. I know that being a woman over thirty in today's society is brutal. You're expected to worship at the altar of youth. But I have built my brand on this one simple truth: The alternative to dangerous anti-aging treatments and procedures is *not* doing nothing. Alongside the hero ingredients I've discussed already in this book, there is a practice that, when done correctly, is the solution you've been looking for. I thought Botox and fillers looked good at first, but eventually I realized my skin wasn't improving. And so, along with the lifestyle changes I made, I investigated

---

12. Murphy, H. (2024). "Imaging of woman with facial fillers prompts questions about whether they actually dissolve over time." *Radiology Business*. healthimaging.com/topics/medical-imaging/magnetic-resonance-imaging-mri/imaging-woman-facial-fillers-prompts-questions-about-whether-they-actually-dissolve-over-time

the causes of aging over thirty and stumbled upon what has now become the cornerstone of not only my beauty practices, but my life: microneedling. So let's *finally* unpack what it's all about.

CHAPTER 8

MICRONEEDLING AND DERMAROLLING

You picked up this book because you have a desire to take better care of yourself, to empower yourself to learn and do better for your skin. You've taken the time to read, to reflect, to understand this incredible organ and your relationship not only to it but to your own humanity. You are showing up for your skin now in ways you have never done before, and for this, I honor you.

This is the chapter I've been building up to. This was the game changer in my own skincare journey. So without any further delay, let's talk about microneedling and dermarolling. This is where it gets really good.

A Brief Background of Microneedling

First, what exactly is microneedling? In simple terms, microneedling, also called collagen induction therapy, uses a tool with individual stainless-steel fine-tipped needles to make microscopic punctures in your skin. It sounds scary, but the process is incredibly gentle and safe when done correctly. The tiny injuries stimulate your skin to do what it does naturally when faced with damage: repair itself from the inside out. During this healing response, your body boosts collagen production. This is your natural alternative to Botox and fillers that yields results without altering your face. And the benefits? They're incredible.

Microneedling lives up to its hype *every single time*. It's powerful but natural, working *with* your body to do what it does best. Microneedling is used to reduce the appearance of acne scars or atrophic surgical scars; to smooth fine lines and wrinkles while also lifting and tightening skin, making it firmer and more youthful; to even out skin tone and texture and reduce hyperpigmentation, redness, and age spots; to fade and even prevent stretch marks; and to encourage hair growth in thinning areas. And it does all of this without harsh chemicals or lasers. It's truly a wonderful technique. And the best part? It's empowering to use beauty practices that align with your body's natural rhythms and cycles, knowing that you are giving your body and your skin only the best. This is how you age on your own terms.

One of the pioneers of microneedling was Dr. Lance Setterfield. During his time in practice, Dr. Setterfield noticed that the skin around tattoos was usually smoother than the rest of the skin, and this intrigued him. He started using a tattoo gun on knee surgery scars and was amazed at the results. He called this treatment microneedling.

Dr. Setterfield further experimented with microneedling on aging skin, rosacea, acne, and hair loss. He found that it significantly improved the skin texture, reduced redness and rosacea flare-ups, and catalyzed hair growth. The treatment had a profound effect on the lives of many people, and has been gaining popularity ever since. For most of its first two decades, microneedling was practiced in dermatological spaces, and at-home use was discouraged because if done improperly, it led to infection and scars. But now, there is a safe and equally effective way to do the treatment at home.

8. MICRONEEDLING AND DERMAROLLING

At-Home Microneedling: the Dermaroller

I was first introduced to microneedling by a friend who worked at a luxury European spa and was intrigued by its skin-transforming benefits. I started experimenting on my own skin with various dermarollers, which are an at-home, do-it-yourself microneedling tool. I soon realized that most of the dermarollers available to the public were designed very poorly and didn't contain any needles at all. Instead they were cheap disc-style tools made of wheels covered not in individual, fine-tipped, stainless-steel needles, but rather in spokes that widened at the base causing larger and uneven punctures. It's important to know that if the "needles" are not true needles positioned individually in the roller with precise fine tips, they drag across the skin, tearing it rather than micropuncturing it. Dragging, as you can imagine, causes scars and is not the appropriate technique for dermarolling.

Disappointed with the results (and the fake marketing!), I started to literally take the various dermarollers apart to see what was going on inside. (You can watch my YouTube channel, available by scanning the QR code at the beginning of the book, where I actually take apart various dermarollers to show you *exactly* what cheap brands are doing.) I studied the mechanics of dermarollers and researched the history and benefits of microneedling to understand what an effective dermaroller needed to achieve.

In 2017, I designed and launched my very own high-quality, professional-grade dermaroller featuring 192 individually crafted, CE medical-certified stainless-steel needles. It's the highest-quality dermaroller on the market.

Other dermaroller brands build lesser-quality products because individual needles are more expensive and cost the companies more money, decreasing their overall revenue. But a real beauty brand will care about your skin as much as you do and will ensure that the tools you use are of the highest quality. That is the promise of the signature Gin Amber Beauty dermaroller featuring Real Individual Needles®! It is the only one of its kind on the market. You deserve a dermaroller that works *with* your skin—not against it. With this tool, you can feel confident knowing you're giving your skin the care it actually deserves.

*Yes, **You** Can Dermaroll*

Dermatologists want you to believe that this is not something you can do at home, but the Gin Amber Beauty dermaroller proves them wrong time and time again. Dermarolling is not an industry secret; you need no special qualifications. There are steps to follow and correct products to buy, but what I've created is one-of-a-kind and accounts for all of these. This is *not* complicated. And I believe in it so much, I put my name all over it. This is the one tool I wish every woman knew about and felt empowered to explore.

The Gin Amber Beauty dermaroller is available with needle sizes of 0.25 mm, 0.5 mm, 0.75 mm, and 1.0 mm. There's also a 1.5 mm dermaroller, which should be used only on the body, not the face. All of these have my stamp of approval for safe use at home as long as you've watched all of my videos on proper dermarolling technique (scan the QR code for access). I've proven time and again that dermarolling with Gin Amber Beauty dermarollers is *completely* safe *and* effective. All of my clients and customers have found the results they were seeking by implementing my dermaroller protocols into their regular beauty routine.

Now, I know it can be scary to try something new; you're protective of your skin! You might even have suffered trauma from trying new products or procedures—putting your trust in professionals who were more motivated by sales targets than relationships. Not enough exposure is given to these experiences that threaten your safety and security and overwhelm your coping mechanisms. If you live with chronic or debilitating skin issues, and you are promised a solution but end up with worse issues, *this is a traumatic experience*. Since your face is the first thing the world sees (and judges if I'm honest), and you've already spent your life feeling out of control because of your skin, how can a negative experience with a skin specialist or product or brand *not* cause further trauma?

While many companies out there might just be "another beauty brand," I know that every woman who watches my videos or buys one of my products has reached me because something in her life is hurting. She's embarrassed by her skin, afraid of the signs of aging starting to show, fearful of being left or judged or cast aside. Even if she's young, she has grown up in a society

8. MICRONEEDLING AND DERMAROLLING

that is devoted to perfection, and she feels the pressure to oblige. If you live in and identify with the body of a female, I want to offer you a solution that doesn't validate the injustices of society, but empowers you to decide what you want to do, how you want to do it, and to have the courage to know that the brand you are putting your faith in sees this and honors your story and your right to a peaceful relationship with your skin.

Gin Amber Beauty is not just a beauty brand, it's a community of like-minded people who understand this pain and who have found what they have been looking for: *not* a quick skin fix, but a way of living that puts each woman and her skin at the center of her life and her decisions, giving her back the power that beauty culture has tried to take away. Dermarolling is not just another beauty tool; it's an opportunity to heal yourself, even if that means starting from the outside in and discovering along the way that you always had the power to heal from the inside out—you just needed someone to put the right tool in your hand.

What to Expect: Before, During, and After Dermarolling

Now that you're excited about dermarolling, I'm going to walk you through the steps of a session. Proper preparation, technique, and aftercare are essential for achieving optimal results. And for more details on dermarolling at home, go to my YouTube page (via the QR code) and check out my dermarolling playlist. Everything you need to know is there, including a visual demonstration of each step to ensure absolute confidence!

Before

Make sure your skin is thoroughly cleansed and free of makeup. I recommend a double cleanse, just to be sure. You can cleanse your skin with a cleanser of your choice, but remember you should always avoid harsh cleansers or cleansers with fragrances, parabens, or drying alcohols. Pat your skin dry with a clean towel, preferably a towel you reserved solely for your face.

Gin Amber Beauty has developed a ToxicFree Foundation-certified and gentle way to disinfect your skin and your dermaroller—our natural foam cleanser. For disinfecting your skin, apply a pump to your fingertips and gently spread it onto your skin. Allow the foam to remain on your skin for at least one minute to help eliminate germs and residue. It's important to let the foam break down completely, as contact time is vital for optimal results. After a minute has passed, gently wipe your skin with a dry or damp cloth, but do not rinse it off.

For disinfecting the dermaroller, apply two to three pumps of natural foam cleanser to your dermaroller in its case. Let it sit until the foam breaks down completely. Contact time is vital for optimal results in eliminating germs and residue. After the foam has disappeared, you do not need to wipe your dermaroller before using it. Apply two to three pumps of natural foam cleanser again after the treatment to sanitize the tool after use. Once the foam has disappeared, close your case and pack it away for next time to ensure no cross-contamination. You can also watch my YouTube tutorial (available through the QR code) on the right way to disinfect your dermaroller.

During

To begin, with even and light pressure, roll and lift the dermaroller four to five times across the skin in each area of the face. The process of rolling *and lifting*, versus just rolling up and down or dragging the roller across your skin, prevents you from going over the same area too often.

For those new to dermarolling, use the tool for a maximum of one minute per small area of the face. Full sessions, including the entire face and the neck, should typically last between three and five minutes. Approach the process methodically. Set a timer for three to five minutes. During this time, focus on covering all parts of your face and neck at least once. If you finish early and still have time left, feel free to go over certain areas, like the forehead or crow's feet, again, being careful that you don't exceed one minute in any given area. There are videos on my YouTube channel (through the QR code) where I demonstrate this exact technique, so head over there to have a look!

8. MICRONEEDLING AND DERMAROLLING

If you've been dermarolling consistently for more than six months, you can use the tool for a maximum of two minutes per small area and extend your full session, covering the entire face and neck, to about ten minutes.

It's important not to exceed this, as more time doesn't necessarily mean better results. Many people mistakenly dermaroll for too long, which will irritate and dry out your skin. So as tempted as you are to do *more* in the hopes that you will see results faster, resist. Dermarolling doesn't work that way—and neither does your skin. Slower, more consistent practices will yield better results than quick-fix aggressive practices.

For hard to reach places like under your eyes and around your nose, lips, and ears, use a 0.25 mm mini-dermaroller. Gin Amber Beauty has a mini-roller for these exact uses.

After

Once you've completed a dermarolling session, what you do in the next few days can make or break your results. This is where so many people go wrong—not because they don't care, but because they're overwhelmed by conflicting advice. So let me make it simple for you. I've guided thousands through this process, and here's exactly what I recommend.

First, give your skin a moment to breathe. Avoid cleansing for at least four to twenty-four hours post-treatment. After that, stick to a very gentle cleanser. Avoid anything harsh or gritty.

Hydration is your best friend during these first few days, especially between days two and four when your skin is losing the most moisture. Reach for calming ingredients like pure hyaluronic acid, aloe vera, or niacinamide. These will soothe, plump, and support repair without overwhelming the skin barrier.

It's also crucial to avoid strong actives and exfoliating acids for the first twenty-four to forty-eight hours. That means no retinol, vitamin C (L-ascorbic acid), glycolic acid, or benzoyl peroxide. These are wonderful ingredients when used appropriately, but right after dermarolling, they can cause unnecessary irritation or inflammation.

Another nonnegotiable: no makeup for at least twenty-four hours. This isn't about shaming makeup—it's about preventing bacteria from entering those tiny microchannels in your skin. Let your skin rest and heal without interference.

Avoid direct sun exposure. Dermarolling makes your skin more photosensitive, so protect it from harmful UV rays. When you're outside, wear a wide-brimmed hat and sunglasses and use a toxic-free, mineral-based sunscreen with at least SPF 25—and reapply as needed.

Last, say no to sweat. For at least twenty-four hours, avoid exercising, hot showers, saunas, steam rooms, and pools. These activities can invite inflammation or bacteria into vulnerable skin, and prickling sweat can be uncomfortable.

Remember: Less is more. This isn't the time to test new products or overload your skin with too many steps. Think hydration, rest, and protection. When in doubt, give your skin space to do what it's designed to do—heal.

Common Concerns and Misconceptions

Okay, so if microneedling at home with a dermaroller, or even microneedling with a professional, is starting to sound *intense*, let's address some of the common concerns and misconceptions most people have. I get it, tiny needles puncturing your face sounds ... pretty serious. Many people hear the word "needle" and imagine pain and bleeding. It might sound to you like something that belongs in a medical clinic, not in your skincare routine, but when done correctly, microneedling is one of the safest, most effective tools for supporting skin health—at any age.

Pain and Discomfort

Many people worry about pain during microneedling. Depending on the depth of the needle as well as your level of pain tolerance, microneedling

8. MICRONEEDLING AND DERMAROLLING

is uncomfortable but not painful. The sensation afterward feels like a mild sunburn—only mild discomfort. You can use over-the-counter topical numbing creams before your session to minimize discomfort if you have sensitive skin.

Bleeding

A common misconception is that microneedling should cause bleeding. In fact, you should not bleed during or after a proper session. Many people who became our clients had reached out to Gin Amber Beauty for help due to injuries caused by excessive bleeding from initially using other, inferior tools or aggressive techniques. To prevent bleeding, it's recommended to start with a smaller needle size and gradually increase the depth of needles as your skin adapts. Of course, it's not necessary to move to a deeper needle at all unless you're dealing with issues like deep wrinkles or scars. In that case, my recommendation is to start with 0.25 mm and work your way up to 0.75 mm, or 1.0 mm for deeper skin concerns, over a period of one year. Yes, one year! This means that you should consistently use each size needle for approximately three months before moving to a deeper one to ensure your skin has adapted to the practice and limit discomfort or side effects. Remember, your skin is like you—resilient! Repeated, safe exposure to smaller needles prepares your skin for deeper needles. Many people, even professionals, mistakenly begin with larger needles, which can lead to unnecessary skin trauma. Patience and perseverance are key.

Skin Reactions

It's completely normal to experience some redness or slight burning after microneedling. These reactions are usually mild and a sign that your skin is responding to the treatment. However, if you experience severe burning, dryness, or swelling, it's an indication that something went wrong—perhaps you used a needle that was too large or you went over an area for too long.

Make sure to do thorough research, like watching all my YouTube dermaroller playlist videos (which you can access by scanning the QR code at the start of the book), before beginning your journey. There are countless resources available online, including detailed guides and videos that can help you refine your technique. Having all of the knowledge in advance means you will feel confident when you do start! You'll also ensure you avoid any mistakes rather than learning from them. And when it comes to your skin, prevention is better than cure.

Results

It's important to manage your expectations when it comes to the results. While many notice improvements shortly after treatment, optimal results typically appear after several sessions, depending on the concern. Consistency and patience are key. Many people give up because they expect the results to be more dramatic, but regular microneedling is a practice you can add to your *lifetime* beauty routine. The best results occur when you use these tools consistently and with the right skincare products.

Depending on your skin's condition, a 0.25 mm tool can be used once or twice a week; a 0.5 mm can be used once a week; and a 0.75 mm can be used once every three to four weeks. Prepare to include these tools in your long-term beauty routine rather than expecting a once-off cure. The more consistent you are, the better your results will be.

Infection Risks

As with any skin procedure, there's a risk of infection if you do not follow proper hygiene and aftercare protocols. If you're dermarolling at home, you must be sure to disinfect your dermaroller head before and after every use. The Gin Amber Beauty natural foam cleanser is liquid oxygen that 100 percent safely sterilizes needles. It's alcohol-free so it doesn't dry your skin out like most alcohols do. Pump one or two pumps directly onto the head of the dermaroller and wait for the foam to disappear before use. The secret to sterilization is the time the needles are exposed to the sterilizing liquid. If you use alcohol for sterilization, spray it on or pour it over the dermaroller head above a sink. Avoid setting the dermaroller in a cup or glass of alcohol so that the needles don't touch the surface and become dull over time. The convenience of my oxygen foam cleanser is that the time it takes for the foam to break down is the time it takes to sterilize the needles, so you'll know exactly when it's ready! The foam cleanser is also gentle on the needles, ensuring they don't get damaged or blunted, which can compromise effectiveness and safety. Alcohol does work, but it

8. MICRONEEDLING AND DERMAROLLING

can irritate the skin and, with repeated exposure, damage the needles. My foam cleanser is the only one of its kind on the market for dermarolling, so I recommend using it.

Also, don't share your dermaroller with anyone, no matter how nicely they ask! Rather, send them my way for their very own.

The Right Microneedling Tools

When it comes to microneedling, knowing where to start can feel overwhelming, especially if you're looking for quality tools. It's important to understand that not all microneedling tools on the market are created equal. A significant number of the options might not be authentic or safe. In my experience running a microneedling business since 2017, I endeavour to constantly research the latest tools and trends to ensure that what I offer my clients is the best, so I have done my research on them all.

Let's break down the essentials to help you navigate this journey effectively.

Source Quality Tools

If you're based in the U.S., you likely can purchase high-quality microneedling tools online. However, if you're located elsewhere, availability might be limited. Wherever you are, it's crucial to ask the right questions to ensure you're investing in a safe, effective product. The Gin Amber Beauty dermaroller—and the soon-to-be-launched Gin Amber Beauty microneedling stamp—are the highest-quality products on the market, and we ship anywhere in the world! I have many happy clients in places as far away as South Africa!

Check for Medical-Grade Certification

Always look for tools that specify "medical-grade needles." This indicates that the needles are designed for safety and effectiveness. If the product claims to use "real individual needles," it's worth digging deeper to verify this claim. In my experience and investigations, they usually don't. This is why all Gin Amber Beauty products come with verified Real Individual

Needles®, 100 percent stainless-steel medical-grade needles. You should settle for nothing less than this.

Inquire Directly

Don't hesitate to contact customer service for clarification about the needles used in their tools. A reputable company should be willing and able to provide this information.

I frequently receive images from clients who opted for cheaper options, often from online retailers, only to face serious skin damage. Your face is delicate; it's not the same as treating tougher skin on your arms or legs. The consequences of using inferior tools can lead to long-term harm or scarring. While high-quality tools and products are not cheap, it's better to invest in those that actually work than cheaper options that don't. It costs money to source the best ingredients and people to put the best together, so you're buying a guarantee as well. It might feel like a leap of faith investing in high-quality products, but you won't be sorry. And remember: You've worked hard to get here, and you deserve to give yourself the best knowing that what you are doing for your skin is loving and a reflection of everything in your life that has brought you here.

Replacing Your Microneedling Tool

I recommend replacing your tool after every ten uses. Just like a razor blade dulls over time, so does your tool. The less sharp the needles are, the less impactful your results will be. Gin Amber Beauty has dermarollers with replaceable heads so you won't have to buy an entirely new device each time the needles become dull. We do this to ensure our brand is doing its part for the planet while still offering you the quality you expect. Although the initial cost may be slightly higher due to the complexity of the design, you'll save in the long run by only needing to replace the heads. My goal is—and always has been—to provide an affordable, high-quality option for anyone looking to use dermarollers. Remember: You want to see your microneedling tools like any other beauty product; they all need to be replaced from time to time.

8. MICRONEEDLING AND DERMAROLLING

If you're unsure about the effectiveness of your tool, ask yourself how long you've had it. If it's been sitting around for over two years, that might explain why you aren't seeing the results you hoped for.

Proper Disposal

When it comes time to replace your tool, you might wonder how to properly dispose of it. While there are no strict regulations for at-home devices in the U.S., it's generally good practice to dispose of the tool in a safe manner. If your tool offers replacement heads, remove the old needle head carefully and place it in a sharps (thick plastic) container. Then dispose of your sharps container according to community guidelines. For those tools that don't have replacement heads, follow the same procedure but dispose of the entire tool.

Professional Microneedling

Finding a qualified esthetician or dermatologist who specializes in microneedling is an option if you prefer not to do this at home. Here is some essential information to confirm before booking an appointment.

Background Knowledge

Ask about their training and experience. Specifically, inquire about the microneedling books they've read. Many estheticians may have learned basic techniques in school but lack in-depth knowledge! This is what sets Gin Amber Beauty apart: I spent many years doing the research before launching my products.

Technique Awareness

It's vital to understand the difference between various needle sizes and their appropriate uses. If a professional cannot explain this or has not engaged in ongoing education, you may want to look elsewhere. If they use a pen dermaroller, they should use the stamping technique and not drag the tool.

Experience with Products

A well-informed professional should be able to discuss the tools they use, how they perform procedures, and the expected outcomes. They also should explain their tool sterilization process; in a clinic or salon, the risk of infection is higher if the tools are shared between people and not sterilized properly.

No practitioner should be intimidated or irritated if you repeat your questions. If they are, it's a sure sign that they aren't confident in what they're doing, and you should look elsewhere! It's your skin—you know it best, so trust your gut.

A Personal Touch

I understand how the world of skincare can feel overwhelming, especially with so much conflicting information out there. When I first began microneedling, I felt the same way. That's why I'm passionate about sharing my knowledge and experiences. If you have any questions or are considering microneedling, don't hesitate to reach out. I want to make this journey as smooth and effective as possible for you.

Finding the right path can feel scary sometimes, and you may have tried various treatments and products only to be left feeling confused or unsatisfied. In my experiences, I discovered that the true secret to radiant skin lies not in expensive procedures or temporary fixes, but in understanding and nurturing my own body. It also helps to find other women who want to share advice along the way—like me! Visit **ginamber.com** to join the community.

When people see me, they often assume I'm younger than I am. It's not about trying to look like I'm in my twenties; it's about looking vibrant and healthy at any age. That's the goal—to feel confident and radiant in your own skin. I often remind my clients that aging is a natural process; what you really want is to look and feel your best.

Self-care is about more than just aesthetics; it's about nurturing the soul. Too many people chase quick fixes, but that's not the solution. Genuine transformation requires commitment and an open mind.

8. MICRONEEDLING AND DERMAROLLING

Investing in yourself is not just about financial expenditure (and all of its corresponding stress); it's about time and effort. You have to treat yourself like someone you love. It's okay to spend money on things that enhance your life; it doesn't matter whether it's getting your nails done, buying that new dress or serum, or enjoying a nice meal. Don't forget to take care of yourself! You need to give yourself permission to enjoy life and to treat yourself with kindness.

You don't need to spend a fortune to learn about self-care. With a little research and dedication, you can transform your routine and embrace a healthier, more fulfilling life.

Invest in yourself—you have worked long and hard enough for everyone else to have earned this just for you.

CHAPTER 9

ADDITIONAL SKINCARE TOOLS

While the magic of microneedling is my go-to beauty tool, there are others that I personally use and recommend. Each of these tools can be used together with everything I've already discussed in this book, so don't be afraid to expand your beauty practices! Each tool complements and enhances the benefit of microneedling and has its own unique benefits. But, as with everything in this book, knowing why these tools are used for skin health, as well as whether they can work for you, allows you to make decisions about your own personal skin journey. And isn't this simply all you're looking for as a woman?

You've walked the journey this far with me, so by now you know that I always recommend working *with* your skin rather than against it. That's why I always lean into simple, safe alternatives like red light therapy, anti-aging patches, facial massages and yoga, gua sha, and at-home skincare routines with my hero ingredients. They might not deliver overnight solutions, but they support your skin's natural processes which are far more sustainable and better for your health. So what do I recommend?

Noninvasive Tools

LED Light Therapy

Of all the tools I've explored over the years, this is one I keep coming back to, not just for my skin, but for my overall health.

The most well-known light therapy is red light therapy. This works by delivering low-level wavelengths of red and near-infrared light to the skin through LED masks or panels, stimulating cell regeneration and repair. This isn't just about reducing wrinkles; it's a holistic boost to your overall health. Red light therapy heals your skin at a mitochondrial level, and with regular use, it even boosts your immune system. As you age, this kind of support is crucial and energizes not just your skin, but all the cells in your body.

Other light therapies that target different concerns include green light to address pigmentation, blue light for acne, and yellow light to soothe inflammation. This versatility means you get exactly what you're looking for—and they are all perfectly safe for use at home. LED light therapy is extremely gentle; I've used it for everything from root canal healing to reducing pain.

And the best part is that even though it involves light, there is no heat or discomfort, meaning your very delicate skin is protected. All you have to do is sit or lie down and let your skin bathe in the goodness of light! Like with microneedling, light therapy fits into your life, so you're more likely to be consistent in using it, yielding better and longer-lasting results. When you have the power to do something about your skin in your own hands, you'll be amazed to see how much more committed you are.

Anti-aging Patches

Frownies® are my go-to tape for anti-aging! I've tried several brands, but nothing compares to their effectiveness. If you haven't heard of facial tape before, it's a specialized gentle adhesive designed to stick to your skin and reduce movement in areas of your face that normally move quite a lot, like your forehead, around your mouth, and next to your eyes. They train the

9. ADDITIONAL SKINCARE TOOLS

muscles where wrinkles often form to move a bit less. You wear Frownies® at night to prevent moving those muscles while you sleep. They effectively act as a noninvasive alternative to Botox that you can use at your own discretion. At first, wearing them might feel uncomfortable—like having cement on your forehead! But you get used to it. And the results are worth it! After wearing them overnight, my forehead is noticeably smoother. Just warn your partner if you wear one—it can be quite a shock to wake up next to someone with a taped face!

Facial Massages and Facial Yoga

Facial massages and facial yoga are more incredible noninvasive techniques to incorporate into your routine. Both yield similar benefits. While facial massage involves physically touching your face, facial yoga often doesn't.

If you're looking to firm up your jawline, something like a simple oil massage can help. By gently sliding your hands upward along your jawline repeatedly, you're essentially giving your muscles a workout. And the sensation of gently touching your skin is a wonderful way to connect with yourself and show yourself some love! Like all massages, it also releases feel-good hormones, meaning time with yourself *and* a dose of dopamine.

On the other hand, facial yoga might involve stretching techniques that also provide great results. I like to practice facial yoga while I'm doing other things, like waiting at a traffic light. Instead of wasting that time, I'll stretch my face! (If you live in Miami and you see a blonde woman in a Tesla pretzeling her face, it's probably me....)

You'll want to be careful and ideally seek guidance from licensed professionals when exploring these techniques. There's a lot of misinformation out there, so look for credible sources, like licensed estheticians or certified yoga instructors.

Gua Sha

Gua sha is an ancient Chinese technique that involves using a smooth-edged tool to massage your face. It promotes blood circulation and can reduce puffiness while also functioning as both a massage and yoga technique for the face. Just remember to use a light touch and glide the tool gently along your skin, moving toward your neck and armpits to encourage lymphatic drainage. You can find plenty of tutorials online, but ensure you're learning from knowledgeable sources to avoid any harm. I recommend using only stainless-steel tools. With regular use, Gua Sha can feel like a workout for your facial muscles. It's also fantastic to do before dermarolling!

Buccal Massage

If, like me, you're always looking for interesting and alternative ways to promote good skin health and delay aging, then look no further than a buccal, or intraoral, massage. It involves massaging the buccinator, or cheek, muscle from inside the mouth. It's a unique approach to facial massage that's worth exploring if you're looking for something different. I recommend watching some videos online from reputable sources before attempting it yourself.

Interventional Tools

Lasers

Lasers have been a popular choice for the skincare world for quite some time, and for good reason. They promise instant anti-aging and flawless skin, tightening and rejuvenating with little to no pain. But my relationship with lasers is a cautious one. I've seen far too many clients in their forties and beyond who opted for lasers hoping for instant results and ended up with serious side effects. They are also usually very expensive, so if this is an anti-aging solution you are considering, here are the facts.

Lasers are heat-based treatments that are used to stimulate collagen production and tighten the skin. They require very little effort from you and offer immediate results, so why wouldn't you be interested? The problem is that these lasers reach extremely high radiofrequency temperatures that can literally *melt* the fat in your skin. Yes, I said melt. Why does this matter? Because the fat in your skin is exactly what gives your face its smooth, youthful appearance! Once you remove this, your facial structure can actually change, and this can be very difficult to restore. I've worked with women who have come to me in desperation, dealing with hollow cheeks and sunken eyes all because of these "noninvasive" laser treatments that promised to improve their skin. You may even need fillers or fat transplants to restore the structure to your face, which means more money and complications than you signed up for.

Laser treatments often result in red, painful skin and require a long recovery time, which can make them inaccessible for women who can't afford to take weeks off. There are cheaper, safer ways to heal your skin!

Laser treatments are an example of the trauma I discussed in the previous chapter. It can be a very distressing experience to not get what you were hoping for when it comes to skin treatments and tools. I see women all the time who have been deeply wounded—emotionally and physically—by treatments they were pressured into doing or outlandish assurances of safety and efficacy. When you have your power taken away in situations like this, it can leave you feeling very skeptical about any skincare tool or technique that guarantees results and can drive you deeper into hopelessness. So many women who find their way to me have had their trust broken and truly don't know how to heal—not just their skin, but their ability to believe that there is hope for any situation.

Sadly, many women do less research when selecting a skincare procedure than when choosing to buy a car. So be sure to understand what you are signing up for and what you can expect before making a decision. This is how you keep yourself empowered.

Embracing Plastic Surgery

If you are particularly set on getting a more dramatic change, I suggest exploring surgical options like a mini-facelift instead of chronically relying on toxic fillers and Botox or considering laser treatments. Yes, I said go under the knife. I believe that every woman has the right to choose what's best for her, and a once-off surgical procedure can actually be safer than long-term exposure to toxins from Botox and fillers. These procedures are performed by skilled surgeons and typically have less risk of long-term skin damage. With a good surgeon, you can achieve a natural look that enhances your features rather than altering them completely.

Perhaps you didn't expect this from me. I know the nip-and-tuck approach doesn't seem like the kind of advice a holistic esthetician would offer, but remember, everything I have built and believe in is founded on this truth: You have the right to do whatever you want—with your skin, your body, your life. Breaking free from cultural expectations and pressures doesn't just mean pursuing alternative therapies. It means *you have the right to choose*. You also have the right to have access to honest, safe information.

Some women do want immediate results. This doesn't mean that you have low self-esteem or that you are giving into sexist narratives. It doesn't mean you don't love yourself! It simply could mean that because you have spent your entire life trying every little thing on the market without results, you have reached a point where you are after the no bullshit approach. It also could mean that plastic surgery is a way for you to align your face or your body with how you see yourself. Either way, I am here to offer my personal and professional advice: Plastic surgery is a good option for improving your skin's health and appearance. There needn't be any judgment or apology for this. For example, a mini-facelift is a very popular procedure among women over forty. This procedure involves small incisions around the ears and hairline to lift and tighten the skin. It's a more permanent solution compared to lasers and doesn't compromise the skin's protective barrier. While it is an invasive procedure that requires general anesthesia (and these risks should always be considered when you're thinking of plastic surgery), it is less invasive than other procedures and the recovery time is much less.

Finding the right plastic surgeon is crucial. This is the most important advice I have for you regarding plastic surgery. I recommend it as an option on the condition that you use someone highly skilled and highly recommended. It will usually cost more to work with a doctor who is popular, but you can never go cheap with this. I repeat, don't look for cheap when it comes to a plastic surgeon. There are no shortcuts, so don't believe anyone who tells you there are. Look for someone with a strong portfolio of before-and-after photos and positive testimonials. Ask for permission to speak to their clients directly so that you can ask questions and get insight from the person who went through it. You cannot simply trust a photo online or a few words on Google. Due diligence is, in my opinion, a necessity in this case. Then, and only then, when you feel secure in your choice, go for it. Women have spent far too long being told what they should and shouldn't do with their bodies. But remember that being an empowered woman means reclaiming the right to *choose*. Your body is yours.

The Emotional Aspect of Beauty Treatments

Now, I want to touch on something deeply important: the emotional aspect of these decisions. Whether you choose to pursue surgery, lasers, or holistic methods, it should come from a place of self-love, not self-hate. Many people mistakenly believe that altering their appearance will fix underlying insecurities, but that's rarely the case.

I've heard heartbreaking stories of people who underwent procedures thinking it would change their lives, only to feel exactly the same afterward. True transformation starts from within. Working on your mindset, your self-worth, and your emotional health is just as vital as any physical treatment.

Trying to fix your skin with hatred will only create more misery. People do this when they live and see themselves through an extremely critical lens. The problem is that when the "work" is done, the critical self view remains. This is the relentless pursuit of perfection. It leads to always finding error and fault in everything; and I can assure you that no surgery or procedure can fix this. When they say that "perfection" is the highest form of self-abuse, they are not wrong.

In the end, it's all about balance. While there's no shame in wanting to enhance your appearance, it's essential to ensure that these decisions align with your values and promote your well-being. Loving your skin and treating it with care can be incredibly rewarding. The best part? You don't need to rely solely on high-tech solutions. Like this chapter has shown, simple routines, mindfulness, and a bit of patience can go a long way.

My message for you is that self-care *is* a form of self-love. Whether it's through light therapy, facial massages, or even more significant changes like surgery, the motivation should always be to make beauty choices that align with your values, protect your body, and leave you feeling like *you*. True beauty—internal and external—comes from that place of love and acceptance. You deserve to embrace who you are as a Divine Woman, and the right tools, whether they're holistic methods or advanced therapies, can help enhance that beauty. Every decision you make in your skincare journey should empower you. If it does, then it's always the right decision.

A NOTE FROM ME TO YOU

I want to say from the deepest part of my heart—thank you. Thank you for walking this journey with me, for being open, curious, and brave enough to reclaim your health and beauty from the inside out. It's no small thing to take your healing into your own hands. I celebrate you. And I am so proud of you.

Writing this book was never just about skincare. It was about truth, freedom, and learning to love yourself without toxins, filters, or shame. I've been where you are. I've felt the confusion, the frustration, the overwhelm. That's why I created this space—for people like you and me who want something deep, real, and honest.

You don't have to do it alone. I'd love to stay connected with you, hear about your wins, and support you through your setbacks. My inbox is always open. Reach out. Tell me what resonated. Share your story, your progress, your glow.

Join my community on YouTube, Instagram, TikTok, or Facebook, and visit **ginamber.com** for more resources, tools, and support. You'll find a whole world of people just like you—learning, healing, and growing together.

This is just the beginning.

With love and light,

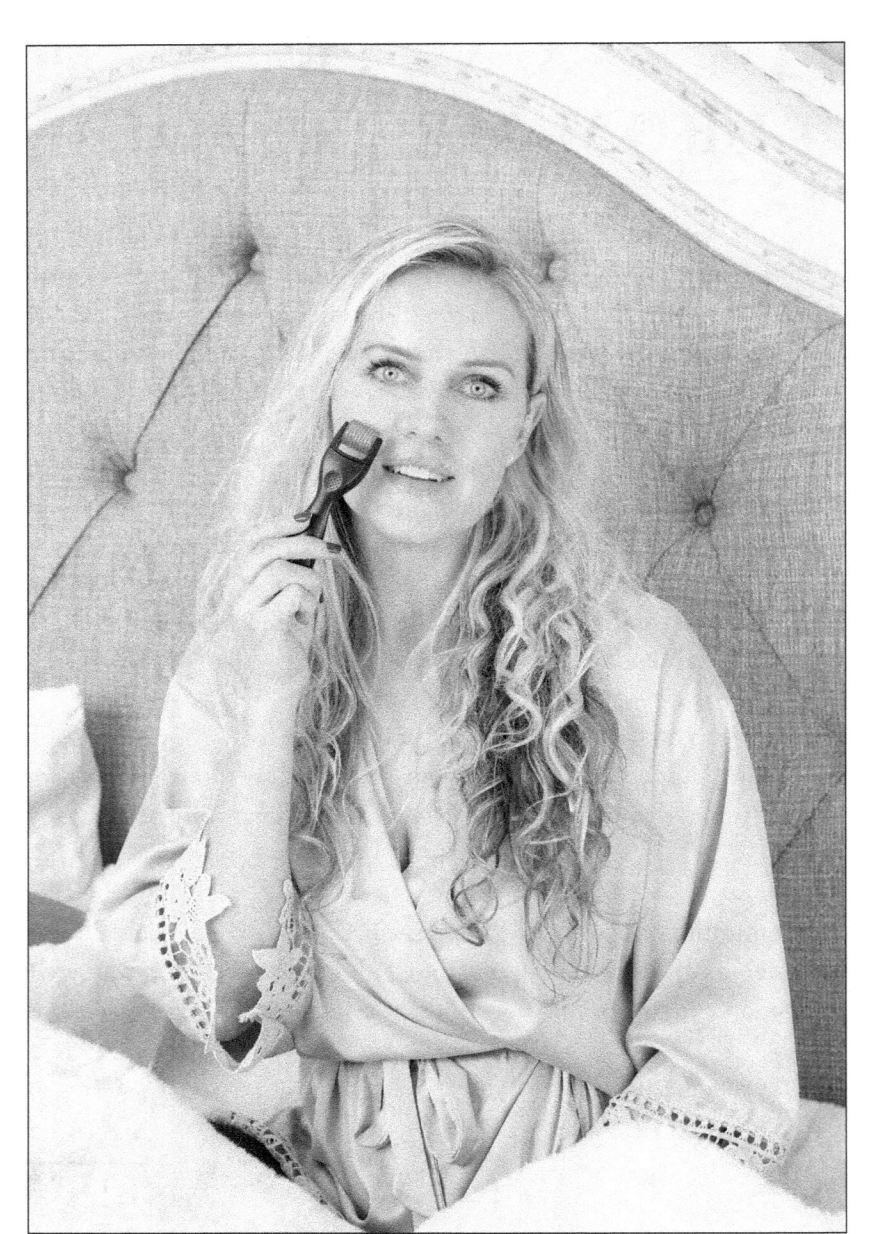

ABOUT THE AUTHOR

GIN AMBER has spent the past twenty-five years immersed in the skincare and wellness industry—not only as a seasoned professional but as a woman who has walked the path of self-healing. After facing a series of autoimmune conditions that left her exhausted and disconnected from herself, Gin was guided toward a deeper journey of healing—one that included nutrition, nervous system regulation, trauma recovery, detoxification, and a return to natural, toxic-free living. For the last fifteen years, she's worked hands-on as a holistic esthetician, combining ancient wisdom with modern science to help clients restore their balance, radiance, and confidence.

Today, she leads a global community of over 500,000 across YouTube, Instagram, and TikTok, inspiring others to reclaim their health and beauty from the inside out. As the founder of Gin Amber Beauty, her passion led her to create a microneedling brand and clean skincare line focused on real, visible results like firmer skin, reduced wrinkles and scars, and a youthful glow without invasive treatments. Her tools and teachings are about making professional-grade care simple, accessible, and grounded in the highest form of authentic self-love.

Through her work and this book, Gin hopes to help others—especially women—reconnect with their bodies, calm their symptoms, and draw closer to God. Because true beauty begins the moment you choose kindness toward yourself.

To connect with Gin and learn more about her work, please visit https://**ginamber.com**.

FREQUENTLY ASKED QUESTIONS

How often must I replace my dermaroller?

We strongly recommend using the dermaroller (any size) no more than ten times. With each use, needles naturally become dull. For optimal results, you want the sharpest needles possible to properly stimulate new growth. That's why there's a checklist on our dermaroller boxes, so you can mark off each use and easily keep track.

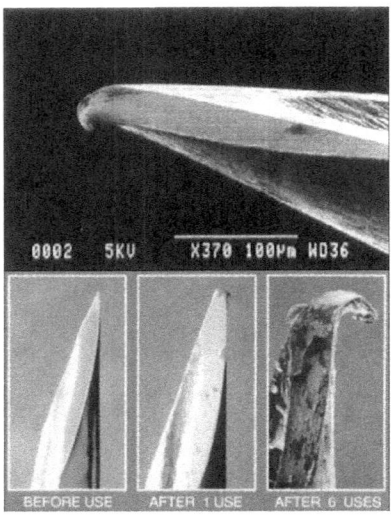

How long should my dermarolling session last?

If you're a beginner, limit your session to no more than five minutes, including the neck area. If you're advanced (have used the dermaroller for more than twenty sessions), you can extend it up to ten minutes.

Can you tell me which dermaroller is best for which kind of treatment?

Selecting a size will depend on your skin type, experience, and the result you're trying to obtain. However, a general rule is to always start with a smaller size like the 0.25 mm dermaroller to help your skin ease into the treatment.

Find your right size by taking a personalized assessment at **ginamber.com**.

FREQUENTLY ASKED QUESTIONS

Are your needles made out of stainless steel?

Gin Amber Beauty dermaroller needles are made of surgical stainless steel, which is why they are so sharp, making dermarolling safer and more efficient.

Does the dermaroller come with a protective case?

Yes, it comes in a plastic protective case and is sealed in hygienic wrapping for your safety upon first use.

Is dermarolling painful?

With proper execution and use of a real dermaroller, it's not as painful as it seems! Using real dermarollers creates even punctures rather than tears that harm the skin, meaning guaranteed results through continuous use. However, do note that the deeper the needle size, the more likely it is to cause discomfort. But you can minimize this by applying a numbing cream.

How do I disinfect my dermaroller and my face before dermarolling?

Because alcohol dries out the skin and heavily disrupts its protective lipid barrier, we no longer recommend using it. Instead, we've developed a certified ToxicFree® and gentle natural foam cleanser to disinfect the dermaroller and your skin.

For your skin, apply one pump of the natural foam cleanser to your fingertips and gently spread it onto your skin. Allow the foam to remain for at least one minute to help eliminate germs and residue. It's important to let the foam break down completely, as contact time is vital for optimal results. After one minute has passed, gently wipe your skin with a dry or damp cloth, but do not rinse it off.

To disinfect your tool, apply two to three pumps of the natural foam cleanser to your dermaroller. Let it sit on the open case and allow the foam to break down completely. Contact time is vital for optimal results in eliminating germs and residue. After the foam has dissolved, you do not need to wipe your dermaroller. Apply two to three pumps of natural foam cleanser again after the treatment to sanitize the roller after use.

What can I expect after my session?

Slight redness, dry skin, and a mild tingling sensation are typical reactions after dermarolling. The longer the needle, the longer these effects may last due to deeper skin penetration. In general, redness should diminish within twelve hours, and the tingling sensation should subside within twenty-four hours. Keep your skin hydrated while it heals using Gin Amber Beauty advanced hyaluronic acid serum.

Will dermarolling cause bleeding?

Bleeding is extremely rare with Real Individual Needles® dermarollers, thanks to the precise, fine needles and carefully selected depths. While minimal pinpoint bleeding may occur with longer needles, especially on areas where the skin is thin or close to bone, most users experience none at all. This is in sharp contrast to wheel-style dermarollers, which are more likely to cause unnecessary trauma and bleeding due to the use of fake needles.

What are the best products to put on my face after dermarolling?

Always consider what to apply after dermarolling because not only is your skin more sensitive, the products can also affect the healing process. Our serums (except retinol), creams, and sheet masks have been specifically developed to be safe to use after dermarolling. Each has its own targeted benefits but can also work together to boost efficiency and overall improve your skin's appearance.

FREQUENTLY ASKED QUESTIONS

If you choose to use other brands, please make sure the products don't contain toxic or irritating ingredients such as fragrance/parfum, parabens, phthalates, SLS, or drying alcohols.

After dermarolling, how long should I wait before washing my face or applying makeup?

This depends on the size of the roller that you used. With a 0.25 mm and 0.5 mm dermaroller, you can do it the next morning or after at least twelve hours. With a 1.0 mm, it is recommended to wait a full day, twenty-four hours.

Why must I follow the guidelines?

It's crucial to adhere to the instructions provided by your practitioner if you receive your treatments in a clinic or my instructions if you are using Gin Amber Beauty tools. Many new users think they can push their limits after the initial experience. However, respecting the guidelines is essential for safety and effectiveness. I emphasize following a structured regimen to maximize the benefits while minimizing risks.

Remember: Patience and consistency are key!

How long will it take before I start to see results?

Microneedle therapy is a long-term, cumulative process. Permanent reduction in wrinkles and scars occurs when new collagen and elastin are stimulated and new skin is generated. You'll usually see results within four to eight treatments, though some may notice improvements as early as the next day.

Can I dermaroll if I have acne?

You should never roll on active acne, cold sores, or any raised/patchy skin abnormalities as this could spread and cause infections.

Can I dermaroll if I'm pregnant?

Yes, dermarolling is perfectly safe to do during pregnancy and even while nursing.

Can I use a dermaroller after waxing?

Do not use a dermaroller of any size on recently tweezed, waxed, or threaded areas. These areas are often tender, and rolling on sensitized skin can increase the risk of irritation or unwanted reactions. We recommend waiting at least seventy-two hours before treating those areas.

How long should I wait after dermarolling before swimming?

Swimming, whether in salt water, fresh water, or chlorinated water, can be done safely after seventy-two hours for all needle lengths.

Can I dermaroll if I have Botox or fillers?

Yes, but it is advisable to wait two weeks before or after an injection.

Do you ship internationally?

For our international readers, it's essential to know that shipping availability varies. We ship to most countries, but always check the latest shipping guidelines at **ginamber.com** to ensure you can access what you need.

www.ingramcontent.com/pod-product-compliance
Lightning Source LLC
LaVergne TN
LVHW012114070526
838202LV00056B/5729